Difficult conversations in medicine

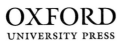

Edited by

Elisabeth Macdonald

Consultant Emeritus, Guy's Hospital, London, UK

OXFORD

UNIVERSITY PRESS

This book has been printed digitally and produced in a standard specification
in order to ensure its continuing availability

OXFORD
UNIVERSITY PRESS

Great Clarendon Street, Oxford OX2 6DP

Oxford University Press is a department of the University of Oxford.
It furthers the University's objective of excellence in research, scholarship,
and education by publishing worldwide in

Oxford New York

Auckland Cape Town Dar es Salaam Hong Kong Karachi
Kuala Lumpur Madrid Melbourne Mexico City Nairobi
New Delhi Shanghai Taipei Toronto
With offices in
Argentina Austria Brazil Chile Czech Republic France Greece
Guatemala Hungary Italy Japan South Korea Poland Portugal
Singapore Switzerland Thailand Turkey Ukraine Vietnam

Oxford is a registered trade mark of Oxford University Press
in the UK and in certain other countries

Published in the United States
by Oxford University Press Inc., New York

ISBN 978-0-19-852774-9

Contents

List of contributors

Author/editor
Dr Elisabeth Macdonald
MBBS FRCR MA
(Medical law and ethics)
Consultant Clinical Oncologist
Consultant Emeritus Guy's Hospital,
London, UK

Contributors
Professor Peter Maguire,
Professor of Psychiatric Oncology,
Christie Hospital,
Manchester, UK

Dr Theo Schofield,
Fellow in Communication,
The Oxford Centre for Ethics and
Communication in Healthcare Practice,
University of Oxford;
Treasurer, Steering Committee,
Royal Society of Medicine Forum
on Communication in Healthcare

Melinda Edwards,
Consultant Paediatric Psychologist,
Guy's and St Thomas Hospital and
South London and Maudsley Mental
Health Trust, London, UK

Liz Martinez, LLB MBA
Solicitor and Medical
Negligence Specialist;
CEDR accredited mediator

Dr Carmel O'Donovan, MB MRCP
Independent Medico-legal
Consultant, Claims Manager
and Risk Management Adviser

Dr Cathy Heaven, SRN PhD
CRUK Psychological
Medicine Group,
Christie Hospital, Manchester, UK

Dr Michael Parker, PhD
Oxford Centre for Ethics and
Communication in Health Care,
University of Oxford, Oxford, UK

Dr Catherine Hood,
Clinical Tutor in Communication,
The Oxford Centre for
Communication in Healthcare,
University of Oxford,
Oxford, UK

Katherine Murphy,
Director of Communication,
The Patients Association

Carolyn Pitceathly,
Senior Research Fellow,
CRUK Dept. of
Psychological Medicine,
Christie Hospital,
Manchester, UK

Acknowledgements

Dr Diana Brinkley for wisdom and friendship.

Professor Peter Maguire for support at the critical moment.

Colleagues and friends at Guy's Hospital, London for education and example.

Lorraine Plummer for the tedious job of typing the manuscript.

Dedications

For Michael Sears, Francesca and Lyssandra.

Preface

The doctor–patient relationship has been evolving over the last few years. Increasing public awareness of health issues and the ready availability of health information both in the press and via the Internet have led the public to be more widely informed about common conditions and the treatments available. Patients therefore come to a medical consultation better informed and more questioning than previous generations.

Public confidence in the health-care professions has been severely undermined in the UK by a series of failures and accidents in an unfortunately wide variety of medical specialities. There have, for example, been concerns about the availability of intensive care beds and the transfer of the severely injured over long distances to these centres, the failure of quality control in cervical cancer screening, the malfunction of cancer treatment machines, the closure of local accident and emergency centres and the disastrous results of heart surgery in children at the Bristol Cardiac Centre leading to the public outcry that resulted in the Bristol Inquiry. Among the many thoughtful and wide ranging recommendations of the Bristol Report is a recommendation that a fundamental change in relationships between health professionals and the public is required based in future on candour and openness, self-analysis and lay involvement. Seventeen of the final 240 recommendations relate to communicating with patients.

In the UK, in response to the public demand for improvement in standards of health-care and health information, the government issued The NHS plan in July 2000. Among the core principles enunciated in this White Paper is the commitment that: 'The NHS will shape its services around the needs and preferences of individual patients, their families and carers'. Among changes envisaged for patients were the greater provision of information in order to empower patients and the strengthening of patient choice. Other profound social changes have taken place within our community. World-wide migration has resulted in the admixture of many cultures and languages in most countries of the world. In parallel with many agencies the medical profession needs to respond to this mixture by adapting the doctor–patient interaction in a manner that is appropriate to the community it serves.

Skill in communication is a matter of personal ability, which varies widely between individuals in the medical profession as in any other. Many doctors instinctively handle difficult conversations well. However, there is always something to reflect on that may facilitate future conversations. Some doctors on the other hand, have not acquired the confidence and sympathy to which patients respond and to some degree this can be learned.

Slowly over the last few years the importance of teaching communication skills has been acknowledged.

In 1993 the General Medical Council recommended that communication skills should be taught at all stages of medical education in the UK. More recently, the Royal

College of General Practitioners has incorporated assessment of these skills into the examination for Membership and other Royal Colleges are following this lead.

In 2001 the Forum on Communication in Healthcare of the Royal Society of Medicine embarked on the process of defining a core curriculum for communication in medical education. This process is well advanced and it is envisaged that this discipline will be incorporated into the medical school curriculum, the doctors' revalidation proposals and the training programmes of the postgraduate institutions over the next few years. (See Appendix II for a copy of the Undergraduate Core Curriculum.)

This book is intended to support this initiative and provide a practical introduction to some of the core principles. It is aimed at doctors and other health professionals in the early years of medical practice to help polish their communication skills and to avoid pitfalls, mistakes or simply embarrassment on either side.

The aim of this book is to dispel the anxieties that contribute to poor communication by describing a relatively simple formula that can be adapted to a wide variety of patients and situations.

Contributors will follow a similar approach bringing their experience of situations and actual formulations of terminology and discussion appropriate to each patient's needs. An overview will be included of the legal framework in which these conversations take place.

In pursuing the analysis of good communication this book places the patient at the heart of this enterprise. As a result the discussion and observations are clearly important for all those who find themselves in the role, at some stage of their lives, of being a 'patient'. The lay public may find it interesting and informative to read a doctor's view of the doctor–patient relationship, an inter-relationship that appears to fascinate the public, yet is not often revealed outside the privacy of the consultation room!

Introduction

Theo Schofield

This book is about the art and science of medicine: the art of the individual doctor or nurse communicating with their patient, and the science of ensuring that this communication effectively meets the patient's needs.

The individual doctor

The principal characteristic of art is that it is an individual endeavour on the part of the author, the painter or the composer. This view of doctor–patient communication was in the past very prevalent. The consultation was regarded as the doctors' domain and under their direction, their abilities were inherent and individual, and substantial variation between doctors was entirely acceptable.

A number of things have happened to change that view. The first is the growing body of evidence that some approaches to communication are more effective at influencing outcomes than others. Patient-centred consulting in which ideas, information and decisions are all shared is more effective than more traditional approaches to the consultation (Stewart 1995). The easiest outcome to measure has been patient satisfaction, what the patient feels after an interview, and importantly in fee for service systems, whether the patient returns to see the same doctor again. Intermediate outcomes include whether the patient becomes less concerned about their problem, whether they adhere to the treatment that was proposed in the consultation and whether they make any changes in life-style or the way in which they respond or control their condition. The ultimate outcome is whether their health improves as a result of reduced concern, adherence to treatment, or life-style change.

The classic series of studies by Greenfield *et al.* (1985) showed by a series of randomized controlled trials that informing and involving patients in their care could produce reductions in blood pressure and improvements in diabetic control that were comparable with the introduction of a new drug. Effective communication was a drug that could be prescribed!

The second challenge to the individualistic view of doctor–patient communication has come from the growing experience that effective communication can be taught and learnt. The majority of effective teaching programmes have three core ingredients: an explicit model of what is to be learnt, opportunities to practice that model and feedback on performance. These models have been informed by the empirical evidence about patient-centred consulting. The opportunities to practise have come either from real patients or frequently from simulated patients and actors, and giving feedback has been greatly helped by the growth of audio and video recording. This experience of effective teaching was summarized in the consensus statement produced at the Toronto conference in 1992 (Simpson *et al.* 1991). This provided some of the support for the inclusion of communication skills as a core recommendation in the UK General Medical Council guidance for medical schools, *Tomorrow's Doctors* (General Medical Council 1993). The elements of good communication that form the basis of many training programmes are described in Chapter 2.

Much of this teaching is provided in separate courses, sometimes by non-clinicians, and therefore remains outside the mainstream of clinical practice (Hargie *et al.* 1998). This does not diminish the quality of the teaching, but can affect the student's perception of its relevance and create conflicts for them between theory and practice. The ward round is a very good example of effective teaching through an explicit model of what is to be done, 'tell me the patient's history', the opportunity to practise by clerking patients and feedback when the history is presented. This has taught generations of medical students to ask questions and to 'take a history' rather than listen to the patient's story. If every case presentation had to include answers to the questions, 'What does the patient think is wrong with them?', 'What are the patient's main concerns?' and 'What would the patient like us to do for them?', we might move a long way towards encouraging more patient-centred interviews. Hearing the patient's story also means that every interview is not just an opportunity to practise skills but also an opportunity to learn about life and illness from one's patient.

It is essential not to lose sight, however, of the role of the individual doctor and in particular their own aspirations, feelings and inherent style of communication. Developing an individual's awareness of these attributes and building on them are an essential part of any effective teaching programme, and unless a doctor can cope with their own feelings, then he will not be able to engage in many of the difficult conservations described in this book. The doctor's perspective and ways of maintaining balance are described in Chapters 6 and 14.

The individual patient

Not only does a doctor need to develop their own individual style of consulting, they also need to be able to vary the style to suit their individual patient. This ability to tailor one's approach to different situations and different people is probably the most difficult to learn and to teach. Many of the difficult conversations described in this book occur when patients are distressed, or when they are of a different age group, educational background or culture from our own.

Each patient has their own ideas about their problem, what caused it and how it could be treated, their own concerns about the implications of the problem for their life, their work and their future, and their own expectations for information and involvement in decisions and treatment. There is a growing body of evidence about the variation in people's belief about health, their understanding of risk, and their desire to be involved in decisions about their care, and the factors that may affect these such as age, or social and cultural background. However, there is an enormous danger that this information can be used to create stereotypes leading us to believe that we already know what a patient's ideas are on the basis of our first impressions, and to fail to explore them in the mistaken belief that this saves time. However, establishing the ideas, concerns and the expectations of the individual patient makes the task of explaining, reassuring and planning management so much easier, as well as so much more effective. David Tuckett and his colleagues described the consultation as a 'meeting between experts' in which the doctor was the expert in diagnosis and diseases, and the patient was the expert in their own symptoms and experience (Tuckett *et al.* 1985). Allowing the patient to tell their story in their own words not only establishes the history but also their language, their explanatory models and their reasons for consulting. Tuckett found that explanations given by doctors that 'reacted' to the patient's ideas and explanatory models were much more likely to be retained than those that did not. Up to 80% of the important information about the problem, its causes and how it could be managed and prevented was retained if reactive explanations were used.

The relationship between a patient and their doctor

Balint in his seminal book, *The Doctor, His Patient and the Illness* (Balint 1957), described the doctor–patient relationship as a mutual investment company to which both parties were committed and on which both parties could draw. He worked with small groups of doctors describing their difficult patients. Many of these were those who, when encountering distress in their lives, presented with physical symptoms, both because they were experiencing them and because these were the symptoms in which they thought their doctor would be interested. He described how these patients could be diagnosed either at a superficial physical level or at a more complex psychological and social level, and how frequently they were referred from doctor to doctor for investigation with no one taking an overview or responsibility for the whole patient, 'the collusion of anonymity'. These patients still exist today and are to be found in every general practitioners surgery, and many hospital clinics, having normal endoscopies, exercise ECGs and CT scans. If all we can offer these patients is medical technology then we fail to meet their needs.

The relationship between the patient and their doctor has enormous potential to be therapeutic if it is based on trust and mutual understanding. This means understanding the whole person, their situation and their concerns, and committing oneself to that relationship and that person. This is more demanding, but also much more rewarding, for both doctor and patient. The science also supports this view. For example, patients with non-organic headache are much more likely to resolve their symptoms if their concerns and worries are discussed when they attend a neurology clinic (Fitzpatrick *et al.* 1983).

Per Fugelli in his Williams Pickles lecture to the Royal College of General Practitioners in 2000 (Fugelli 2001) described the essence of trust as being the belief that the doctor is acting in the patient's best interests. Trust can be earned by honesty, compassion, commitment to the person and their best interests, and by competence. Trust can be undermined by a lack of trust in the benevolence and honesty of the institutions in which we work, and by creating conflicts of interest for the individual such as financial incentives and inappropriate targets. A lack of trust means that patients will be reluctant to share their concerns and their vulnerability, less willing to accept the doctor's advice and reassurance without multiple tests and investigations, and be more demanding and more inclined to complain or sue when things go wrong.

The reason that so many patients are turning to alternative medicine is not just that scientific medicine does not have a cure for conditions such as migraine, back pain or chronic fatigue but also because alternative practitioners give of themselves and their time to understand their patient and to individualize their care. Their treatments may not stand up to vigorous scientific scrutiny, but their care, the 'drug doctor' that Balint described, does.

Medicine in context

Like art, the style of communication between doctors and patients is influenced by the society in which it is practised. The decline in deference and respect for authority that took place in the second half of the twentieth century affected both individual relationships and the relationship between the media and the professions. The availability of information from sources other than health professionals has enabled people to question and challenge them. The ethical and legal framework in which we work has developed to give primacy to respect for autonomy and informed patient choice, rather than beneficence and compliance with medical advice (Chapter 3).

Many of these changes are to be welcomed and provide an opportunity to develop partnerships with patients and to involve them much more in their own care. However, these changes can feel very uncomfortable for doctors and nurses at times, particularly when working under pressure. They have led to more 'difficult conversations', and the fact that this book contains a chapter on how to deal with a complaint and offer an apology, Chapter 13, is a marker of these changing times.

The growth of evidence-based medicine has arguably led to more effective care, more conformity to guidelines and protocols, and greater accountability for practice. It has also produced challenges for communication between doctors and patients, balancing the 'right' answer from the evidence with the patient's perspective and choices, informing those choices in ways that the patient can understand, and sharing power and decisions with patients without losing the ability to make patients feel cared for (Bensing 2000).

The explosion in medical knowledge and technology may have 'fixed' many problems such as infectious diseases and safer surgery, and created much greater patient expectations for cure and a pain-free life. What remains, however, is an older population with more chronic problems requiring care rather than cure. Expert technical care may save the life of a person with an acute myocardial infarction, but this life may then involve psychological adjustment to a new self-image, changes in leisure activities and employment, and adaptations to life-style to reduce the risks of a subsequent event. All these require a supportive and long-term relationship with a number of doctors and nurses over a long period of time.

The development of both high technology medicine and long-term care has meant that much more of it is delivered by teams rather than individual professionals. The abilities to communicate effectively with colleagues and to work as a member of a team are now essential for effective patient care. Some of these conversations may be difficult as described in Chapter 11, but working as a member of an effective harmonious team can also be very supportive and rewarding for the individuals, as well as giving better quality of care for patients.

On the other hand the health-care system in which the individual doctor or nurse works can have a very negative effect on care and communication with patients. The view that the motives of those working in the National Health Service are largely altruistic has been undermined in a society based on consumerism and profits, and by a few highly publicized scandals. The mismatch between demand and expectations on the one hand, and financial and personal resources on the other, creates conflicts for health professionals, and between them and their patients.

It is now recognized that for many aspects of quality improvement in health care it is as important to look at the system and the way it works, as to focus on the individuals working in it. Facilities and care for staff have a low priority in many parts of the National Health Service. This can lead to feelings of being undervalued and exploited, and it requires a high degree of self-awareness and commitment to avoid letting these feelings affect one's attitudes to patients.

Shift systems can increase workload and diminish continuity of care, and demands for throughput can diminish the time available for each individual patient. These pressures are felt most acutely by junior hospital doctors at a time when they are learning their style of communication and their attitude to patients and patient care. It is easy to see how the tender flower of patient centredness sown and nurtured during medical school can wilt and die in the hothouse of the emergency room.

It is therefore very important to equip those individuals with the survival skills required to work within the system. These include self-awareness, the ability to give and to seek support from colleagues, and also the ability to be assertive rather than aggressive under pressure.

Conclusions

This book is therefore about the individual doctor, how you relate to your patient, and how you respond to the society and the system in which you work. Learning core skills and approaches will help to equip you, but learning about yourself and what you want to express in your work, and about the perspective of the patient and how to make that your central concern, will enable you to give real depth to the art of medicine.

References

Balint, M. (1957). *The Doctor, His Patient and the Illness*. Edinburgh: Churchill Livingston.

Bensing, J. (2000). Bridging the gap. The separate worlds of evidence-based medicine and patient-centered medicine. *Patient Education and Counseling*, **39**, 17–25.

Fitzpatrick, R.M., Hopkins, A.P., Harvard Watts, O. (1983). Social dimensions of healing: a longitudinal study of outcomes of medical management of headaches. *Social Science and Medicine*, **17**(8), 501–10.

Fugelli, P. (2001). James Mackenzie Lecture. Trust—in general practice. *British Journal of General Practice*, **51**(468), 575–9.

General Medical Council (1993). *Tomorrow's Doctors. Recommendations on undergraduate medical education*. London: General Medical Council.

Greenfield, S., Kaplan, S., Ware, J.E., Jr. (1985). Expanding patient involvement in care. Effects on patient outcomes. *Annals of Internal Medicine*, **102**(4), 520–8.

Hargie, O., Dickson, D., Boohan, M., Hughes, K. (1998). A survey of communication skills training in UK Schools of Medicine: Present practices and prospective proposals. *Medical Education*, **32**, 25–34.

Simpson, M., Buckman, R., Stewart, M., Maguire, P., Lipkin, M., Novack, D., Till, J. (1991). Doctor-patient communication: the Toronto consensus statement. *British Medical Journal*, **303**, 1385–7.

Stewart, M.A. (1995). Effective physician-patient communication and health outcomes: a review. *Canadian Medical Association Journal*, **152**(9), 1423–33.

Tuckett, D., Boulton, M., Olson, C., Williams, A. (1985). *Meetings Between Experts: an approach to sharing medical ideas in medical consultations*. London: Tavistock.

Chapter 1

An introduction to basics

Elisabeth Macdonald

Summary

Good communication between medical staff and patient is important because it forms the basis of all future health-care transactions. Communication needs to be patient centred and informative. It needs to promote trust and confidence between participants of equal status. Good communication is important to avoid the harm that could ensue in terms of patient dissatisfaction, non-adherence to the advice given, psychological damage, physical harm, litigation or even death. Beneficial effects have been demonstrated on health outcomes and not only patients but health-care workers also benefit from a satisfactory exchange.

Why is good communication important?

Good communication between patients and medical staff is important from the very first encounter because this forms the basis of all future transactions. It sets both the tone and the agenda for the future relationship not only with this individual doctor but also between the medical profession as a whole, other health-care professionals and the patient and his or her family. This first interaction provides the foundation upon which the future relationship will be built. Conversations about health care need to be first and foremost patient centred. The focus of all health care is the individual patient and as professionals we need to be aware that without the patient all our training, effort and expertise is as meaningless as an empty restaurant, tables laid, waiters waiting, chef poised but not a diner in sight!

In primary care the first encounters with a family doctor often suffer from severe time constraints. However, many general practitioners become very skilled at eliciting a wealth of information from a patient with a few well-aimed questions. This may on the other hand 'lead' the consultation according to the doctor's agenda without giving the patient the opportunity to volunteer the real reason for the visit. Patients are frequently left dissatisfied by these short transactions, although it is fair to say that the skill of the doctor may leave patients unaware of how much information they are volunteering. Patient satisfaction does, however, depend not only on being heard but also on feeling heard.

In the hospital environment, whether in the Accident & Emergency Department or in the ward setting, it is very often a junior doctor or nurse who is the first health-care professional encountered by a person who may have had no previous experience of ill health or the complex world of professional health care. It is therefore incumbent upon the junior staff to establish an effective relationship with both patients and families, which will promote trust and confidence throughout the patient's future progress. Junior doctors also usually represent the members of the medical profession with whom patients have most frequent contact throughout their hospital stay. Consultants and senior members of the medical team spend most of their time in the operating theatre, the outpatient clinic or the laboratory. As a junior doctor you are an essential member of the team so don't be apologetic! You are the vital conduit of information on ward issues between staff members and between patients and staff.

At first sight this initial conversation appears inherently problematic. Two unknown quantities, the doctor and the patient, meet on uneven, unknown ground often with little common background, in a situation that requires them to share information. The patient on the one hand has his own unique perspective derived from personal experience, education, knowledge or ignorance of health topics, culture and family background. The health-care professional on the other hand comes to the meeting with a certain level of general education, specific professional training, often until now little training in communication skills and variable natural common sense in personal interactions.

The objective of a successful consultation is to enable these two participants to conduct a one to one conversation of equal status. The doctor needs to 'tune in' to the patient and remember that different phrases mean different things to different people.

In later conversations the doctor may well be delivering information, which the patient really does not want to hear. This means of course that the information is news that the patient would prefer was not relevant to him or her. However, having accepted that it is relevant the patient will want to know the full picture. This conversation needs to build trust and to establish a shared approach to the patient's problems. Such conversations are not a single interaction but represent a process, which may take time and require revisiting and re-enforcement on many subsequent occasions. None the less in appropriate circumstances a few succinct short phrases can be very useful. Some of the most critical conversations need not in fact take a long time. A few words of the right kind at the right time can make an enormous difference to the morale of a frightened or depressed patient. Whatever the circumstances the aim is to establish and maintain trust and a shared approach to the patient's problem.

Good communication is vital from the outset, not only to establish good rapport but also to avoid the harm that can ensue from failed communication. Unsatisfactory conversations can lead to many negative outcomes principally for the patient but also in fact for the clinician.

Potential harmful consequences of poor communication

The patient who feels denied the opportunity to explain his concerns may feel alienated, frustrated, resentful or angry. Patient dissatisfaction can lead ultimately to non-adherence to treatment advice, to frank psychological morbidity, physical harm, litigation and at its worst the patient's death.

Negative feelings aroused by poor communication can lead on to rejection of the proposed management plan and the potential loss of opportunities for health improvement. Non-cooperation in therapeutic measures may result in poorer outcomes than could have been achieved and adverse events that could have been postponed or avoided altogether if a satisfactory doctor–patient relationship had been established. In many diseases not only the quality but also the timing of medical care is vital. Early diagnosis and successful intervention can, for example, abort the natural evolution of many forms of cancer in the early stage. Poor communication at a critical moment, which fails successfully to recruit the patient's aid and cooperation, may needlessly give time and opportunity for a tumour to metastasize and kill. Diabetic complications can to some extent be prevented by early life-style changes if the patient's cooperation is enlisted at an early date.

Some research work has been done to evaluate the influence of communication on health outcomes (Kaplan *et al.* 1989).

Stewart (1995) for example described the numerous overall benefits that can be observed after a satisfactory consultation. These include a reduction in concern or anxiety levels and the lessening of distress. Health and functional states were seen to improve and there was better control of symptoms such as discomfort or pain. Objective measurement demonstrated a lowering of blood pressure.

In a further analysis Stewart *et al.* (2000a) in Wisconsin, Canada observed improved health status and increased efficiency of care with a reduction of diagnostic tests and referrals when family physicians implemented patient-centred consultations.

Similarly in a systematic review of the therapeutic effect of the doctor–patient relationship, which included 11 medical, psychological and sociological electronic databases, Di Blasi *et al.* (2001) reported the consistent finding that physicians who adopt a warm, friendly and reassuring manner are more effective in therapeutic terms than those who keep consultations formal and do not offer reassurance.

All patient groups clearly benefit from this approach but older patients in particular respond well when their expectations of a sympathetic consultation are met. Good quality communication with the elderly was found to improve recall of the conversation, adherence to the advice given and patient satisfaction. In outpatient visits the development of a continuing relationship seemed to be important in decreasing the necessity for hospitalization among older patients (Stewart *et al.* 2000b). In all these studies it was the success in establishing common ground between clinician and patient that was identified as the most important fundamental.

Patients are not the only beneficiaries of good relationships. Doctors and nurses in today's hectic world gain enormously from the interest, warmth and emotional satisfaction of effective communication with patients and their families. Generosity of purpose guides most clinicians and the pleasure of a difficult job well done brings contentment and fulfilment to the true professional. And don't forget the power of laughter to defuse a tense situation or relax the anxious worrier! Humour needs to be included with care but in the right circumstances and at the right time a smile and a joke can reassert normality, a flash of warming sunshine across an otherwise gloomy horizon.

Potential harmful consequences of poor communication

- Patient dissatisfaction
- Alienation
- Frustration
- Resentment
- Anger
- Non-adherence to treatment
- Psychological morbidity
- Litigation
- Accelerated death

References

Di Blazi, Z., Harkness, E., Ernst, E., Georgiou, A., Kleijnen, J. (2001). Influence of context effects on health outcomes: a systematic review. *Lancet*, **357**, 757–62.

Kaplan, S.H., Greenfield, S., Ware, J.E., Jr. (1989). Assessing the effect of physician-patient interaction on the outcomes of chronic disease. *Medical Care*, **27** (Suppl. 3), S1 10–27.

Stewart, M. (1995). Effective physician-patient communication and health outcomes: a review. *Canadian Medical Association Journal*, **152**, 1423–33.

Stewart, M., Brown, J.B., Donner, A., McWhinney, I.R., Oates, J., Weston, W.W., Jordan, J. (2000a). The impact of patient-centred care on outcomes. *Journal of Family Practice*, **49**(9), 796–804.

Stewart, M., *et al.* (2000b). The influence of older patient physician communication on health and health-related outcomes. *Clinics in Geriatric Medicine*, **16**, 25–36, vii–viii.

Chapter 2

Fundamentals of good communication

Elisabeth Macdonald

Summary

This chapter analyses the important elements of good communication. This involves both initiating and responding skills and is an interactive process both giving and receiving information. Helpful techniques are explored, including the use of active listening, non-verbal encouragement and response to cues. Physical surroundings and practical arrangements are discussed. Linguistic aspects of the consultation are analysed, including the role of language and the structure of the consultation in a sequence of phases. Effective time management is vital and suggestions are given to help keep the conversation on track and to deal with the garrulous or the reticent patient.

Elements of good communication

Communication is an interactive process. From a doctor's point of view it involves both initiating and responding skills. A great deal of the eventual effectiveness of medical management depends on eliciting accurate information from the patient. Good history taking is an art that forms a fundamental part of medical education and is an indispensable tool of good medical practice. Much of the information required is factual and, therefore, it is essential that the doctor lead the patient through focused relevant questioning in order to ensure that important facts are established and that no relevant practical issue is neglected. This traditional type of 'history taking' has long been taught as a core skill in medical training. In this type of interview the framing of simple intelligible questions is fundamental. In general the principles of history taking cover a history of the current complaint in sequence, with dates, to establish the nature of the problem that has brought the patient to seek medical advice. Then follow details of past medical history, family history, social enquiry, drug history and allergy enquiry. Of equal importance, and hitherto neglected in history taking, is the establishment of the patient's perspective on the interview, his own ideas, concerns and expectations. In abbreviated terms some refer to this information as 'ICE' (ideas, concerns and expectations). In exploring the patient's agenda you should involve patients in the endeavour to find common ground. When it comes to discovering this less tangible information then a more productive approach can be one of active listening, open-ended questioning and appropriate response.

Serve your history with ICE (ideas, concerns and expectations)

Conversations in primary care, outpatient clinics and in hospital

Conversations between doctor and patient take place at various stages of the patient's 'journey' along their medical pathway. Conversations in primary care tend to elicit new health-care problems and concerns that may vary hugely across the spectrum of health and disease. They can involve such widely differing topics as influenza, pregnancy, injury, depression, backache, impotence or eczema. Outpatient consultations on the other hand tend to relate to a more limited area of enquiry depending on the department to which the patient is referred, dealing with either physical or psychological issues. Inpatient conversations tend to be more disease specific. All of these consultations, however, need to encompass the general as well as the specific. Broader perspectives are involved in medicine at every stage and a successful consultation with each doctor will need to reflect this. The art of good communication depends on creating an interchange that satisfies the needs of both participants by actively giving and receiving information in both directions.

Active listening

In conversation we are all aware that the messages we receive result as much from what our eyes perceive as what our ears actually hear. Active listening involves listening with both eyes and ears. Communications researchers have calculated that a very small proportion of meaning in any communication is conveyed by the words themselves. Although a newborn infant has no formal vocabulary few of us would deny that there is plenty of communication when he is hungry or in pain! Researchers estimate that the proportion of meaning conveyed in adult conversation divides roughly as follows: words, i.e. what is actually said (5%); tone of voice (35%); and body language and non-verbal communication (60%). This means that as a clinician if you do not register the body language of the speaker you are potentially missing the real meaning of their communication. In patient consultation whenever you sense a mismatch between words, tone of voice and body language, it is the non-verbal communication that is undoubtedly conveying the truest message. It is hard for anyone other than a professional actor to control or manipulate body language successfully. With effort and self-control we can modulate our tone of voice, but to project, for example, relaxed self-confidence while feeling tense and restless is difficult in the extreme.

When talking to patients it is therefore important consciously to observe their body language. This helps us to focus on what is being said, which can be difficult because speech is inevitably delivered more slowly than thought is processed. If attention is not consciously paid to non-verbal communication then important clues about a patient's real agenda can be missed. Restless activity, for example of the feet and hands, can betray unease and anxiety not conveyed by a patient's speech.

Most importantly the converse is also true. Patients who are aware that the doctor is actively focused on the person in front of them are much more likely to be forthcoming and relevant. Negative body language such as avoidance of eye contact, fidgeting with a pen or notes or the failure of concentration is readily detectable to an anxious patient and is not at all conducive to a productive exchange. In contrast, patients who feel that they have a doctor's undivided attention and are being listened to seriously, will feel that they are valued, that their ideas and feelings are being given due consideration and that they are significant in their own right. On the other hand, don't look too concerned, sad or serious as you may worry the patient even more! Developing the art of active listening will reap an invaluable harvest for all health-care professionals.

Why do doctors find it difficult to listen? Life in medical practice is undoubtedly busy. Many issues and activities vie for attention and action. It is all too easy to become distracted by alternative concerns when we should be concentrating on the matter in hand. We may find ourselves unable fully to listen to what a patient has to say because we are planning what to do next. We may be contemplating the implication of what is being said, we may be disagreeing with the content or we may be rehearsing our reply. We may be anticipating what is coming next and often we seek to hurry the patient on to the next topic. We may be trying to talk at the same time. We may be bored by information that we think is irrelevant and simply withdraw into ourselves. Very often doctors interrupt before the patient has finished speaking, frequently with a further question. Many problems arise because the doctor is simply not listening to the patient's perspective. Apart from the discourtesy that inattention portrays it is important to be aware of having interrupted your listening so that you know when there is the possibility that you have missed something important: 'I'm sorry, I missed what you said there. Would you mind saying it again?'

We may equally well be uncomfortable, too hot, sitting uncomfortably or simply be too tired to maintain concentration. Some doctors just don't think that what patients have to say is of much interest. Herein lies the first step on a perilous path to arrogance and a catalogue of complications.

Encouraging a useful contribution from the patient is an active skill. Encouragement can be given non-verbally with a smile or a nod or by simple expressions such as 'I see'. Repetition of the last phrase or sentence can encourage the patient to continue, while summarizing or repeating what you have heard confirms that you have been listening as well as understanding and encourages further communication.

Positive pauses can be helpful to let the other person relate what they want to say, rather than what you want to know. In active listening mode it is wise to minimize your use of questions. Every time you ask a question you dictate the agenda. This is perfectly allowable when you are checking facts but less helpful when you wish to convey real interest in the other person's viewpoint.

When patients or relatives are having difficulty expressing their feelings it can be helpful to reflect these feelings and volunteer a suggestion such as 'It sounds as though you found this very distressing?' or 'You must have found this rather worrying?' Such a suggestion may 'legitimize' the patient's emotion and encourage them to elaborate. On the other hand, an inexperienced listener who misjudges the emotion or the patient's readiness to confess to it may damage the rapport that had already been established. Most patients will appreciate your effort to be understanding even if you are a bit wide of the mark.

Active listening can prove an invaluable tool in fraught circumstances. When feelings are running high and the patient is voicing anger and distress, it can be very productive to affirm your interest with positive silence. The patient is given free reign and is able to express themselves and their agenda to their own satisfaction. Most angry people tend eventually to run out of steam. By active listening their anger is defused. Eventually, at an appropriate moment, the active listener can respond with an appropriate comment such as 'Okay what would you like to do about it?'

One technique to encourage patient communication, which is frequently employed in the psychological and psychiatric specialities, is that of silence. Positive, receptive and encouraging silence is a further non-verbal stimulus for the patient to continue. This can be a useful means of reaching out to the shy patient who finds it difficult to engage.

Active listening

- Look
- Nod
- 'I see'
- Repeat phrase
- Summarize
- Pauses
- Minimize questions
- Reflect feelings

Physical surroundings

Most conversations can be facilitated by congenial surroundings. In the medical context, this means that where possible conversations should take place in a quiet, private and if possible light and airy environment. The provision of a quiet space away from the hustle and bustle of ward activity or a busy outpatient clinic is helpful wherever possible.

To get the best out of a consultation the doctor should arrange to give single-minded attention to the individual patient or family. This requires a situation to be engineered in which interruptions can be kept to an absolute minimum. Phones ringing, bleeps sounding and other staff enquiries can all unsettle, annoy or distract patients in such a way as to irritate them or destroy a train of thought. The intimation of private or personal thoughts is easily aborted by an inappropriate phone call. Making not only time but also space for the patient conveys respect for their individuality and the importance of their personal information and opinions.

In making provision for useful conversations it can be helpful to encourage the patient or relative to bring with them a friend or family member. This witness to the proceedings can be very helpful in providing emotional support and encouragement to the patient. They can corroborate information and provide a source for checking factual information. Often consultations involve the interchange of large quantities of information and it can be very difficult for the patient to recall all that he or she has been told. When the consultation involves distressing news, it is very common for the patient to fail to register anything other than the one important upsetting piece of information throughout the entire conversation. In these circumstances the presence of a friend can not only provide emotional support but can retain information that would otherwise be lost. They can also provide continuing liaison for the future development of communication with the patient.

The tape recording of conversations for similar reasons is examined in Chapter 10.

Your own personal setting can facilitate easy flowing conversation. A relaxed and comfortable arrangement between two individuals promotes natural and informative interchange.

Some patients feel that the doctor's desk represents a barrier between the two, especially when the doctor buries his head and his attention in the notes placed on the desk between them. A more receptive arrangement can be that with chairs placed facing each other but at a slight angle to reduce the impression of confrontation. Leaning slightly forward or in the direction of the patient implies sincerity and interest while maintaining an open posture conveys confidence. Sitting with knees tightly crossed and especially with the arms folded across the chest, implies a defensive, superior or unhelpful attitude. Try not to look too concerned or too serious! The patient may become overly anxious. Both parties are likely to be more comfortable in chairs that have arms. Mental comfort is more likely to be engendered by physical comfort in which both parties can be relaxed but attentive.

When consulting in an office consider the positioning of the computer screen. If the screen is facing you but away from the patient this can imply a lack of openness. If the screen is at 90 degrees to you both you can share information. If the screen is behind you it will be necessary to break off the conversation to check results and this could be helpful if it gives the patient an opportunity to gather their thoughts.

Eye contact with the patient is extremely important. This does not imply that you should fix the patient with a constant gaze, but regular eye contact throughout the conversation implies confidence and trust. The patient is much less likely to feel that their views are being ignored or that information is being concealed when eye contact is regularly maintained. On the other hand some shy patients are likely to be more comfortable when the gaze is not too steadfast, and reticent patients are more likely to volunteer information if at a particularly difficult moment for the patient the doctor is sensitive enough to look away or drop his gaze. Information, which the patient may regard as private, embarrassing or even shameful, is more likely to be volunteered in a discreet rather than a confrontational setting. Remember also to be aware that eye contact in some cultures especially with members of the opposite sex may be thought disrespectful. Be sensitive to cues of discomfort from the patient.

Listening should be active yet relaxed. Overintense concentration can be intimidating. It is better to cultivate a courteous but quietly confident style. However, an apparently relaxed attitude leaning far back in a chair with the arms behind the head is to be avoided. The doctor may think that this conveys relaxation and openness. On the contrary, this position implies an attitude of extreme superiority and converse to the usual assumption is adopted when an individual, often male, is feeling threatened!

Linguistics

Structure of the consultation

Increasing awareness of good communication in the doctor–patient relationship has promoted academic analysis in this field. (Linguistics = the study of language.) Such work has sought to clarify, quantify and define some relatively intangible aspects of personal interactions, which are difficult to characterize and measure. Derived largely from academic study in psychology and psychiatric medicine this discipline has developed a specific terminology. In particular, there has been study of clinicians' behaviour during medical interviews. There is a growing body of evidence that suggests clinicians use 'individual, distinctive and describable types of behaviour or interactional strategies' to conduct consultations and in particular four components of behaviour have been identified (Frankel and Stein 2001). These components are described as 'habits'. They comprise the opening strategy of the interview, the method of eliciting the patient's agenda, the demonstration of empathy and some important elements of the final phase of the interview. These components bear a partially sequential relationship and are thus interdependent. They reflect and complement the structure of the consultation that is described below in four phases. They thus offer an efficient and practical framework for organizing the flow of medical visits and each component or phase demonstrates families of interviewing skills. These aspects of conversation analysis may be concurrent or sequential. For example, empathy is as demonstrable in the early phase as in the concluding negotiation.

- First phase agenda
- In-depth discussion
- Formation of plan
- Final phase

Other writers have identified what is described as clinical 'hypo-competence' (in other words deficient skills) in this area and have highlighted issues such as inattention to primary symptoms, incomplete patient-centred history taking, a highly controlling style, and failure to form a late working hypothesis (Platt and McMath 1979).

Some of these analytical skills are demonstrated in the Appendix to this book.

First phase of the medical interview (agenda)

Increasing importance is placed on the early phase of the medical interview especially in outpatient consultations. Determining the patient's major reasons for seeking care is of critical importance for a successful medical encounter. Increasingly, emphasis is laid on the importance of establishing the patient's agenda and list of priorities. Hence there is a necessity to use open-ended questions at the beginning of a consultation. This allows the patient to describe the principal problems in his own terms. Open-endedness initially allows one to gather some potentially rich data, helps to develop rapport and to identify the key areas of concern for the patient. These patient-determined issues need to be addressed if the patient is to feel satisfied with the interview even if these do not end up as the primary focus of concern from the clinician's point of view. Some examples of open questions follow:

'What would you like to discuss today?'

'What brings you to see me today?'

'What is it that's been bothering you?'

Some questions on the other hand can be so open as to be unhelpful, e.g. 'Tell me about yourself.'

Some very short open questions can sound accusatory in the wrong context; for example, if a patient describes something they have done or said and you respond 'Why?', this may sound antagonistic. It would be wiser to soften the inquiry with an expression such as, 'What was in your mind when you did (or said) that?' Some further examples of open questions:

'Tell me, how can I help?'

'How are you feeling?'

'How do you feel about . . . ?'

'Are you comfortable with . . . ?'

'Can you tell me about your main problems/difficulties/symptoms . . . ?'

Too direct questioning early in a consultation may make the patient passive and close off the disclosure of important information that could have assisted diagnosis and management decisions. Alternatively, if the patient is not encouraged to list all his concerns it may be only on conclusion of the interview, when the patient has his hand on the doorknob, that he raises a vital issue. This demonstrates that an important matter, possibly the most important issue of the entire interview, has neither been divulged by the patient, nor solicited by the doctor, earlier in the exchange. This is unsatisfactory for all concerned and faces the doctor with the difficult dilemma of pursuing this important issue and delaying other patients or postponing the investigation of this matter until a future visit. (See Final phase of the consultation below.)

Asking about how patients feel in both a physical and an emotional sense will help them open up. Confronting obvious emotional stress early is helpful.

'Are you OK?'

'You seem very unhappy today. Can I help?'

This gives the patient the opportunity to be honest about what is really troubling them. Similarly, with an anxious patient, deal with the anxiety first and try and get it out of the way, 'You seem rather anxious today. Can you tell me why?'

It may be that the concern is ill founded and can be cleared up quickly, 'No, you will not need an operation for this problem.' On the other hand legitimate concerns are immediately identified, 'Well, yes, cancer is one possibility but there are others and that's what we are here to find out.'

Mention of a cancer fear incidentally is very common and should be dealt with straight away. When any possibility exists that malignant disease is present this fear should be acknowledged. False reassurance, later to be disproved, is destructive of trust. If possible, other potential diagnoses (infection, gout, etc.) should be listed, and this is reassuring. Affirm that your intention is to find out what is causing the problem and take action. Agree that this is a legitimate concern and suggest that it was a very positive suggestion to voice this worry now. Wherever reasonable affirm that should this kind of cancer prove to be the problem then there is plenty that can be done about it. Reassurance that is appropriate is the key to future successful navigation of the problem.

In the past, many doctors have received no training in communication skills and have not been skilled at eliciting the full scope of a patient's agenda. Research indicates that physicians frequently choose a patient problem to explore rather than determining the patient's full spectrum of concerns (Marvel *et al.* 1999). This study shows that, although most physicians (75%) did enquire about patient concerns, these initial statements listing problems were only fully completed by the patient in 28% of interviews. Doctors tended to redirect the patient's opening statement after an average time lapse of 23 seconds. It is interesting, and in practical terms helpful, to note that those patients who were allowed to complete their statement about their list of concerns used a further 6 seconds on average only compared with those who were redirected before completing their list.

Another interesting line of enquiry is to establish the predictive value of the presenting complaint, i.e. the first issue to be raised by the patient in a consultation. Burack and Carpenter (1983) investigated the relationship between the presenting complaint and the principal clinical problem identified during new patient visits in an academic primary care setting. They investigated the frequency with which patients start the consultation with the issue that in reality troubles them most. Complaints and problems were classified by content as somatic (physical symptoms or problems), psychosocial or health maintenance. The presenting complaint was correctly identified in 76% of somatic (physical) problems but only 6% of psychosocial principal problems. Doctors were apparently poor at facilitating an exchange in which the patient felt able to discuss sensitive issues of a personal, psychological or sexual nature. This work indicates that, although the presenting complaint is often of importance, it is not necessarily the issue which is most troubling the patient. Quite often it appears that patients may feel that psychosocially sensitive topics are not appropriately shared at the outset of the consultation. The patient may well prefer to withhold a major concern until he or she has enough confidence in the doctor to volunteer this information. Closed questions and early focus on the first reported complaint may prevent the patient raising this, their principal anxiety, at any stage of the consultation. For this reason it is important at later stages of the interview when rapport has been established to check the patient does not have further concerns that need to be addressed.

Some patients have hidden reasons for consulting their doctor. Obviously, the principal reason that brings the patient to the doctor or hospital is the need for medical diagnosis and treatment. However, some also seek help for less obvious reasons and doctors, especially in primary care, need to be alert to alternative motivations driving some patients to seek medical help. Some patients, especially those who are socially unsupported, may seek solace in medical attention following upsetting personal experiences or episodes of social isolation. Some may seek emotional support during a psychiatric disorder or manifest a desire for inappropriate health information (Barsky 1981). Cancer phobia may be one example.

Some patients may seem unduly troubled by their symptoms. Their description of symptoms may seem out of proportion to the possible explanations. Asking the patient what they imagine to be causing their illness may make the visit more intelligible: 'This problem is clearly bothering you. What do you think could explain it? What do you imagine is going on here?'

It may well be that the patient has not volunteered the whole story and needs gentle persuasion to be forthcoming. Perhaps quite separate and possibly non-medical issues such as marital disharmony or job insecurity are at the basis of their difficulties.

Alternatively, when the act of making a medical diagnosis and reaching what seems to you, the doctor, to be a satisfactory conclusion does not appear to satisfy the patient, you should ask the patient how he had hoped you might help. The patient may have an altogether different agenda from that which first appeared. Only a further opportunity to speak their mind will enable some patients to get to the heart of the matter.

Patients who express dissatisfaction with their medical care should be questioned further. They may be dissatisfied because their real motivation in seeking care has not been illuminated. For reasons of lack of privacy or perceived uncertain confidentiality the patient may have felt unable to talk freely and feel that the consultation has been 'wasted'. Active listening may help but just occasionally there are people whose wishes can never be satisfied, who may not know themselves what is really wrong, and who can monopolize a doctor's time to no benefit to either party. Once you have done your best to empathize and to clarify the problem it is legitimate, for the sake of your other patients to end the interview with an offer to see them again when they have had time to think through what it is they feel you can help with: 'I can see we have not got to the bottom of things for you today. I'm afraid we must leave it there but I will be happy to see you again on another day when you have had a chance to think about it a bit more.'

Lastly, patients who initiate a visit but do not actually have any specific physical or psychological complaint may in fact be manifesting a response to some stress in their life and demonstrating a cry for help in their inability to cope with personal problems: 'You seem to be quite well in yourself really but is there something else bothering you?'

Second phase of the consultation: in-depth discussion

The next phase of the interview requires the varied skills of facilitation.

Some patients need to be prompted to continue by comments such as 'Mmm', 'I see', or 'go on'. These may appear to be inert observations but are actually facilitating the confiding of all the patient's concerns. Alternatively take the direct approach: 'How did that make you feel?'

Further encouragement can be given by repeating part of the patient's contribution. These statements can prove effective in prompting further disclosure and do encourage the same topic to be continued but on the other hand can restrict inclusion of the patient's other concerns and prevent the patient completing his whole agenda. Likewise, elaborative questions such as 'tell me more about' encourage pursuit of a single topic in depth but can exclude others. Closed questions limit responses and options much more tightly, whereas some 'non-question' comments such as 'that sounds serious' can encourage elaboration with further helpful information.

This type of linguistic analysis forms the basis of training in the use of communication skills (see Introduction). Beckman and Frankel (1984) have analysed the effect of these linguistic devices on the collection of useful patient information. Seventy-four complete visits to the primary care internal medicine unit at Wayne State University were audio-taped and transcribed between July 1980 and June 1982. Overall, only 23% of patients completed their personal agenda during the visits. The relationship of interruption to subsequent completion of the patient's agenda is most striking. Once the doctor had interrupted the information stream it was virtually impossible for the patient to express fully the reasons for seeking medical advice. Inevitably this leads to 'a dissatisfied customer.' In all these encounters the interruption marked the transition to doctor-centred direct questioning.

Among the linguistic devices used by the doctor to redirect the interview, closed questions were most frequent (46%). In some conversations (12%) interruption occurred before a single concern had been expressed. In all of these consultations it was a return visit by the patient that led the doctor to refer back to previous complaints without waiting to establish whether the patient was coming for a different reason altogether. Interruption moves the focus of information gathering from patient-centred to a doctor-centred format. This treats the patient's first concern as necessarily the most important and as we have shown this is not necessarily the case. Burack and Carpenter (1983) showed that there was frequently a disparity between the patient's chief complaint and the doctor's determination of the principal problem. This underlines the importance of re-soliciting additional concerns throughout the visit.

This research also throws light on the frequent problem of pressure of time in consultation. On average interruptions occurred between 5 and 50 seconds following the doctor's first request for information. In contrast most completed statements took less than 60 seconds and none longer than 150 seconds. Characteristically, after a brief period of time (mean 18 seconds) and most often after expression of a single concern, the doctor took control of the visit by asking increasingly specific closed questions that effectively halted the spontaneous flow of information from the patient. We can conclude, therefore, that giving the patient one or two more minutes to list his problems at the start of the discussion will reap dividends in saved time talking 'off the point' and facilitate a much more productive use of time later in the interview.

Response to cues

Most serious conversations in life contain layers of meaning and when discussing matters of importance we tend to flag up some peripheral issues by means of phraseology or expression. We lay out 'cues' to the listener often in the hope that they will pick up on the issue and inquire further. Some of these are fairly obvious. If we are quiet and withdrawn with little to say we may expect our audience to pick up on this and ask us 'What's the matter?' If we volunteer that we are feeling depressed and worried we expect our companion to ask why. Some cues are more subtle relying on the fact that our friends or family know us well.

Similarly, in consultation many patients give their doctors cues as to their true concerns and feelings. Cues may be in search of either informational or emotional support. Doctors on the whole tend to be better at responding to informational cues than to emotional prompts (Butow *et al.* 2002). One of the main aims of current training in communication skills is to help doctors learn to 'tune in' to their patients and respond to these cues. The skill lies in picking up on cues and reflecting them back. Some responses to cues:

'Are you all right?'

'What's up?'

'Tell me more about . . . . '

'You say you have been worried . . . . '

'What effect does this have on you?'

'You said you thought this might be serious. What did you think might be the matter?'

'I sense that . . . e.g. I sense that you are not quite happy with the explanation you have been given. Is that right?'

'I got the impression that . . . . but now realize I am wrong. Could you tell me exactly?'

'I can see this is distressing for you. Would you like to come back to it later?'

'You say X . . . but while you are talking I feel Y . . . '

Third phase of the consultation: management plan

The third phase of a consultation is in effect the 'business' phase. Now there is an opportunity to complete closed questions of relevance concerning past history, family history, social enquiry, known allergies, etc. Physical examination will often throw important light on the complaint even when this seems from the history unlikely.

The next task is to work with the patient to generate a problem list and decide how best to proceed. A priority list is helpful: 'What bothers you most?'

The next step in the process should be organized there and then if at all possible. Appointments for specialist opinion can at least be requested. Blood request forms can at least be selected etc. In this way the patient has confidence that not only is there an agreed plan of action but that it is being taken seriously.

Closing phase of the consultation

Communication research has also stressed the importance of the closing stages of the interview, both from the point of view of patient satisfaction and outcome effectiveness. Ideally this phase should provide a final opportunity for other concerns to be raised, should restate the management plan and ensure that this is both agreed and fully understood. Arrangements should be made for the next visit so that the patient has confidence that current problems can be reviewed and other issues addressed if necessary.

Research shows that it is usually the doctor who closes down the interview (White et al. 1994). However, only 75% of doctors in this study clarified the future plan for care and only 25% asked the patient if they had more questions. Patients introduced new problems, not previously discussed, in 21% of the 'closures'. This is unsatisfactory and it is not surprising that these new problems tended to emerge following consultations that had been lacking in one or more important components such as attention to emotional or psychosocial issues and a failure to check on understanding.

Satisfactory closure can often be assisted by giving the patient 'warning' that the consultation is nearing an end: 'We have about five minutes left and I would suggest . . . Is that alright?'

Such an intimation that time is nearing an end may precipitate the patient into mentioning something important that they would have regretted omitting. If the patient does not realize that the interview is nearly over they may be left dissatisfied and angry when they do realize they have run out of time.

Occasionally patients may seek to prolong their interview by volunteering an important piece of information right at the end of a consultation. You need to be firm in response to this ploy and ration your time fairly for the sake of your other patients: 'I'm afraid we have, as I explained before, only 20 minutes today and we have taken up our time with your other concerns. Please make another appointment in the near future and I will be happy to explore this matter then.'

Time management

Time constraints in the modern National Health Service are frequently severe. If the health service is viewed simply as a 'Health Factory' through which the maximum number of patients must be processed in the fastest possible time then it may be felt that talking to patients is a luxury. However, this is far from the pattern that the government, the health professions and patients' representatives are seeking to create. If the Health Service is viewed rather as a system in which good health is promoted and patients' needs are best satisfied then the doctor–patient consultation will be seen as pivotal in maximizing these aims.

Whatever the philosophical view of both primary and hospital practice, there can be no doubt that professional time is at a premium. Balancing the need to ration your time fairly between individual patients and between clinical activity and administrative tasks is a real challenge for most doctors.

How can we, when talking to patients, balance the need to work fast with a need to fulfil our obligation to listen to the patient and address their agenda? Many doctors think that if they enquire about the patient's agenda, especially if this involves psychological issues, then the doctor will lose the 'initiative' and the interview will take too long. In reality, the opposite is usually true. Focusing from the start on the patient's most important problems will enable the doctor to use time most effectively.

One way to deal with this problem is to clarify at the start what time you have available: 'What brings you to the doctor today? We have about 10/20 minutes to deal with your most important concerns. If we don't manage to cover all of these then we can come back to them later. Is that all right? Where would you like to start?'

Giving patients a time frame helps them structure their agenda and reassures them that there is time to deal with important issues. Secondary issues may have to wait but the choice of topics is theirs. Patients don't expect their doctor to 'fix it all' in one session but they need to know that the doctor understands that there are other matters to be dealt with and will respond in due course.

This approach, stipulating the time available, although realistic can seem rather defensive and controlling and may not be comfortable for all occasions.

Alternatively, in different circumstances a few seconds or a very few minutes can sometimes be all that is needed to deal with a crucial issue in a timely manner: 'I am due in the outpatient clinic in 5 minutes but the ward sister tells me that you have a new pain. Could you tell me about it and we can arrange some X-rays this afternoon and get them reported by the time I do my round this evening?'

The patient understands that the doctor is busy but will be reassured that the health-care team is communicating among themselves and that new problems will be speedily dealt with.

On the other hand a patient may take the lead. He may not want to repeat the same story for the tenth time but would prefer to deal with the priority matter. This view should be respected. If there are many problems ask the patient which is his priority and deal with this first.

Much depends on the attitude and style of the patient. In order to gain maximum benefit from their consultation with the doctor patients can make sensible preparations. Working out in advance the points to make and if necessary preparing a list can facilitate a productive exchange. This topic is further addressed in Chapter 5. People vary in their ability to convey their meaning, and different personalities respond in different ways to the anxiety engendered by the medical environment. Some people become withdrawn and inexpressive while others become anxious and garrulous. Putting the patient at his or her ease will relieve anxiety and help to keep the conversation on track. Different skills are needed to draw out the shy patient or to focus the garrulous patient and the development of these techniques is rewarding in both a personal and a time-management sense.

Garrulous patients

When voluble patients get carried away with their account of things you may need to practise some techniques to persuade them to stop talking! Your body language may help. Shifting in your seat or shuffling your notes may indicate you want to move on.

Pick up a word of import and repeat it to divert the flow in that direction: 'Pain. Oh I see, you had pain. Tell me about that.'

Interrupt and explain why your next question is important and then ask it. Be assertive and not aggressive: 'Sorry to interrupt but it is very important for me to be clear about the sequence of events. Did you have this cough before you developed a temperature?' In a sympathetic way you could also interrupt and say, 'I can see that event upset you but we don't have very long. Can we come back to that later?'

Alternatively, give the consultation a structure, a framework and a time scale and say you will deal with problems at the end: 'What I suggest we do in the next 10 minutes is hear what happened to you in the accident yesterday, then I would like to examine you and arrange some X-rays. Is that all right? We can come back to your rash later.'

Alternatively you could say 'I'm sorry to go on about this but I really need to know . . . . '

Then again you could try and get into the patient's underlying agenda by asking, 'What do you think it is?'

Used carefully some of the following phrases may help you to keep the garrulous patient relevant. After a lengthy digression: 'Yes, I'm sorry you had that experience but can we go back to . . . ' (this kind of digression is ruefully known as a 'war story'!), or 'Have we exhausted that topic?/I think we may have exhausted that topic, shall we go on to . . . ' This approach will indicate that the information given is probably not likely to be helpful especially if more of the same is on offer.

Some questions anticipate a very definite response and can help navigate through a consultation: 'Have you finished what you wanted to say?' implies 'Yes', and that you think that the patient has indeed finished.

You will find that plenty of opportunity presents itself to practise these techniques!

Reticent patients

Drawing out the shy or reticent patient can also require time and patience and needs a rather different approach. The tone needs to be low key and unchallenging. The aim is to tune into the patient's style and mood. If withdrawn patients are to disclose their problems this will only take place in an atmosphere of trust (Maguire *et al.* 1993). You may elicit more information if you stay quiet and practise 'active listening' as described earlier in this chapter. Sympathetic body language and vocal tone convey your interest.

The shy patient will need to be led gently through the interview with plenty of clarification. Obvious emotion should be confronted and addressed: 'Are you all right? May I ask what's troubling you?' Alternatively, if you are having difficulty eliciting the patient's agenda you could ask a specific question and then open out the conversation from there: 'Can you tell me when you first noticed this lump and how you found it?'

Pick up on any cues the patient does give you and reflect them back: 'You seem to be very concerned about this lump and not want to talk about it much. Can you tell me what you think it could be?'

Sometimes it will help simply to ask the patient to expand on what they have told you: 'Tell me more about . . . '

Occasionally, patients remain inaccessible and rapport is very hard to establish. What can you do to help this situation? You could begin by acknowledging the difficulty you are having in trying to establish a dialogue with the patient: 'I would like to talk to you today to find out if you are having any problems we can help you with. However it seems we are having difficulty getting into conversation.' In this way the interviewer acknowledges that this is a problem between them rather than due only to the patient (Maguire *et al.* 1993).

Some people are normally very quiet or shy and it may simply take longer to gain their trust and earn their confidence.

On the other hand there can be temporary factors responsible for this behaviour. Anger, distrust, hidden fears, shame or guilt can all manifest themselves as withdrawal. To identify the reasons for this reaction it is important to negotiate carefully to see if the patient is willing to disclose his or her difficulties: 'Can you bear to tell me why you are finding it difficult to talk to me just now?'

The phrase 'Can you bear to . . . ' is a very useful opening described by Maguire for use in many troubled situations when you wish to express empathy within your question.

Some severe manifestations of withdrawal result from depressive illness or psychiatric disorder, and in these circumstances specialist psychiatric help should be sought.

References

Barsky, J., 3rd (1981). Hidden reasons some patients visit doctors. *Annals of Internal Medicine*, **94** (4 Pt 1), 492–8.

Beckman, H.B., Frankel, R.M. (1984). The effect of physician behaviour on the collection of data. *Annals of Internal Medicine*, **101**, 692–6.

Burack, R.C., Carpenter, R.R. (1983). The predictive value of the presenting complaint. *Journal of Family Practice*, **16**(4), 749–54.

Butow, P.N., Brown, R.F., Cogar, S., Tattersall, M.H., Dunn, S.M. (2002). Oncologists' reactions to cancer patients' verbal cues. *Psycho-Oncology*, **11**, 47–58.

Frankel, R.M., Stein, T. (2001). Getting the most out of the clinical encounter: the four habits model. *Journal of Medical Practice Management*, **16**(4), 184–91.

Maguire, P., Faulkner, A., Regnard, C. (1993). Handling the withdrawn patient—a flow diagram. *Palliative Medicine*, **7**, 333–8.

Marvel, M.K., Epstein, R.M., Flowers, K Beckman, H.B. (1999). Soliciting the patient's agenda: Have we improved? JAMA, **281**(3), 283–7.

Platt, F.W., McMath, J.C. (1979). Clinical hypo-competence: the interview. *Annals of Internal Medicine*, **91**(6), 898–902.

White, J., Levinson, W., Roter, D. (1994). 'Oh, by the way . . . ' the closing moments of the medical visit. *Journal of General Internal Medicine*, **9**, 24–8.

Chapter 3

The ethics of communication

Michael Parker

Summary

It is widely recognized that effective communication skills are essential to good medical practice and that communication skills training is a crucial aspect of the training of good doctors. This chapter points out that in addition to being effective, communication must also be ethical. It introduces doctors to core ethical concepts and to the main approaches in medical ethics and shows how these relate to communication in the consultation and to the nature of the doctor–patient relationship. The chapter aims to give doctors a framework for thinking about ethics in communication that will enable them to feel more confident in their consideration of the ethical aspects of their practice. The chapter argues that a necessary condition for ethical communication is that it respects patients as 'persons'. The chapter goes on to explore what this might mean in practice and describes four scenarios which present particular ethical difficulties in communication.

Introduction

The day-to-day practice of medicine requires not only the making of scientific and technical judgements, but also judgements of value. These may be explicit, such as when, for example, a doctor reflects on her own moral views about the permissibility of abortion. Often however, value judgements in medicine are implicit in what might appear at first glance to be 'clinical' decisions. Doctors may not always think of themselves as making value judgements, for example, when considering what would be in an incompetent patient's 'best interests'; when weighing up whether harm to a third party is sufficiently 'serious' to justify a breach of patient confidentiality, or when assessing 'quality of life' in intensive care. Nevertheless, it is clear that these decisions do indeed involve the making of value judgements. Good medicine requires that value judgements such as these are properly analysed and assessed, just as scientific and technical evidence should be properly evaluated and 'evidence-based'. Doctors must be prepared to justify their decisions both with regard to the scientific basis of the decision, and the ethical values by which it is guided. Evidence-based medicine requires interventions to be justified on the existence of evidence for the intervention's effectiveness, and not on other grounds, such as the fact that it is traditional practice, or on the authority of the clinician. What would it mean for a value judgement to be evidence based?

The assessment of value judgements may require several different approaches. These might include comparison of the decision under consideration with those made in other cases, to ensure consistency. They might also include the clarification of key concepts, such as, for example, 'best interest'. It is sometimes also useful to focus on the logical structure of the arguments for and against different options. This will involve consideration of both the truth of the claims being made to support an argument, and of whether the claims, even if true, do in fact support the conclusion claimed for them. That is, whether the argument is 'valid'.

When faced with difficult problems in medical ethics it can sometimes also be useful to stand back and consider the issue in the light of different moral theories. The 'application' of such theories will not usually produce a solution to the problem at hand, neither will it always produce consensus. This is because ethical issues often (but not always) arise for the very reason that there is a conflict between fundamental moral principles, or because different people place different weight or value on these principles. Even in such situations however, the consideration of ethical theory in medical ethics is of value for at least three important reasons. Firstly, it can help doctors to clarify the ethical issues underpinning a difficult decision. That is it can clarify the 'ethical landscape' in which the decision is being made and make it clear what underlies differences of opinion. Secondly, the systematic use of ethical analysis can help to ensure that doctors have reflected on the full range of relevant ethical considerations. Thirdly, it can enable doctors to feel confident that they have made decisions they are able to justify in terms of ethical values, as well as in terms of scientific and technical evidence. Such justification will often involve acknowledging the counter arguments to one's own position.

Ethical theory

Consequentialism

Suppose that as a doctor you are dealing with a case that raises a number of difficult ethical issues. You are considering several possible courses of action and want to know 'which is the morally right course of action?' According to consequentialism, the way to answer this question is to consider the consequences of each of the possible courses of action. An action is right according to consequentialism if, and only if, it promotes the best consequences. This is because, for consequentialists, only the (foreseeable) consequences of an action are of moral relevance. This has a number of interesting implications. It implies, for example, that the question of whether or not lying to patients is morally wrong depends, not upon some features of lying itself, but upon the foreseeable consequences of lying. A consequentialist argument against lying might emphasize its implications for the doctor–patient relationship, or perhaps for trust in the health service more widely, but would not argue that lying was wrong regardless of the consequences.

By itself, 'consequentialism' is an incomplete moral theory. This is because whilst it requires us to base moral decisions on a consideration of which option is likely to lead to the best consequences, it does not tell us which among the possible consequences is morally relevant. For this reason, 'consequentialism' is in fact a cluster of moral theories, differentiated by the importance they place on different types of consequence. Utilitarianism is probably the most influential consequentialist moral theory in medical ethics. Utilitarianism was developed by two nineteenth century British philosophers, Jeremy Bentham and John Stuart Mill. According to utilitarians what is morally important in decision making is the promotion of human happiness and the minimizing of human misery. For a utilitarian confronted by the question, 'which is the morally right course of action?' the answer is the one that leads to the greater sum of human happiness. This is an approach to ethics that will often have a natural appeal for health professionals. The concern to benefit patients and to avoid causing them harm (often referred to as the principles respectively of 'beneficence' and 'non-maleficence') is at the core of what most health professionals consider good practice. In practical terms, what utilitarianism means for ethics in the clinical setting is that when faced by a difficult ethical decision, particular attention should be paid to the foreseeable harms and benefits of each course of action. In fact, for a utilitarian, this is all that is of moral significance.

Duty-based ethics

Virtually all moral theories consider the consequences of our actions to be of moral significance but whereas consequentialists hold that *only* the consequences of our actions have relevance there are other (non-consequentialist) theories that consider other features of our actions to be of importance. One such family of ethical theories is made up of those emphasizing the moral importance of 'duties'. Such theories are often called 'deontological' (from the Greek *deon*, duty). Deontological theories emphasize the duties we have to one another, for example the duty not to lie, and tend as a result to argue that (at least sometimes) even if lying has the better consequences it is still morally impermissible. What such theories have in common, in contrast with consequentialism, is that they consider there to be features of acts (such as lying) that are of moral significance in their own right, irrespective of their foreseeable consequences. According to such theories the question, 'which is the right action to take?' is to be answered by a consideration not of the consequences of possible actions, but of the moral nature of the actions themselves (which may of course include a consideration of their consequences).

Just as there are different forms of consequentialism, different deontological theories will emphasize the importance of different kinds of duties. Some theories will emphasize religious or traditional duties. Others will emphasize duties based in the use of reason. Perhaps the most influential deontological theory of this kind is the secular moral philosophy of Immanuel Kant. Kant argued on the basis of reason for a single moral rule (a categorical imperative) from which all others must be derived if they are to be justified. The categorical imperative was formulated in a number of different ways by Kant. One of the best known of these formulations is as follows,

> So act that you use humanity, whether in your own person or in the person of any other, always at the same time as an end, never merely as a means
>
> (Kant, 2001 (1785))

This formulation of the categorical imperative demands that we respect 'humanity', that is, ourselves and other persons, as rational beings (as 'ends'). To treat someone as an end, is to respect their right to make decisions about the way they wish to live their own life. It perhaps requires too, that we should whenever possible actively encourage the development of the rationality both of ourselves and others. It is easy to see that an approach of this kind is going to place great emphasis on our obligations to respect the choices of others and hence not to deceive or coerce them—even if better consequences (e.g. less harm) could be achieved by even a small deception. In medicine this would suggest the need for a great deal of honesty and high standards of informed consent in the doctor–patient relationship. As with the consequentialist perspective, this form of deontology is likely to resonate strongly with the ethical intuitions of doctors and other health professionals. For it places a great deal of importance on respect for patient choice (sometimes referred to in medical ethics as respect for patient autonomy) and on the need to treat patients as people in their own right. This is also an approach that requires us to stand back from our dealings with individual patients and consider the wider implications for the autonomy of others. That is, it implies an important and central role for a principle of justice, requiring us to respect the autonomy of all patients in for example the allocation of health care resources (such as time in the consultation).

In practice health professionals will tend to draw elements from both of these ethical perspectives. This is one reason why we experience ethical conflict. Most of us would consider it wrong to lie to someone simply because this is likely to lead to the best consequences. But most of us would also find it possible to imagine situations in which telling the truth would have such awful consequences that it would be right to lie.

Principles of medical ethics

Consequentialism and duty-based ethics are general moral theories. It can sometimes be useful when confronted by a difficult ethical decision to step back and consider it in these terms. It is not always necessary to consider medical ethics at that level. Sometimes it is useful to consider decisions in terms of some less abstract ethical principles. One framework of principles of this kind, often used in medical ethics, is the so-called 'four principles' approach developed by Beauchamp and Childress (Beauchamp and Childress, 1994). The four principles they identify are: respect for patient autonomy; beneficence (promotion of what is best for the patient); non-maleficence (avoiding harm); and, Justice (see box). Consideration of a clinical decision in terms of these four principles can be a useful way of sketching out the moral landscape of the decision.

Four principles of medical ethics

Respect for patient autonomy

Autonomy is the capacity to think and decide, and to act freely and independently on the basis of these thoughts and decisions. The principle of 'respect for patient autonomy' requires health professionals to help patients make their own decisions and to respect those decisions, even if the health professional disagrees with them. Helping patients with decision making requires for example, the provision of all relevant information. The principle of respect for autonomy requires us to start with the question 'what does the patient want?'

Beneficence—doing what is best for the patient

The principle of beneficence emphasises the moral importance of benefiting patients. It entails doing what is best for the patient. In most cases the principles of respect for autonomy and of beneficence will require health professionals to do the same thing, because most of the time patients will want what is in their best interests. The two principles will most often come into conflict when a patient chooses a course of action that is not considered, by the health professional, to be in his or her best interests. This of course raises the question of who should be the judge of what is the best.

Non-maleficence—avoiding harm

The principle of non-maleficence states that health professionals should not harm their patients. In most situations, this principle does not add anything significant to the principle of beneficence because the principle of beneficence requires us to weigh up the benefits and harms of all possible interventions as part of the process of deciding what is in the best interests of the patient. Most health care interventions carry at least some risk of doing some harm. This does not mean that they should be avoided but it does mean that the harms of an intervention should be commensurate with the potential benefits.

Justice

The principle of justice requires us to be fair in our treatment of patients. Resources such as the time of health professionals is not unlimited and decisions have to be made about how much time, for example, to spend with different patients. The principle of justice requires health professionals to treat patients in similar situations equally and, when making decisions about the availability of health care resources for one patient, to take into account the impact on other patients.

The need for ethical communication

It will be clear from all of this that communication in the doctor–patient relationship will be of particular interest to medical ethics, whether for consequentialist or deontological reasons. In what remains of this chapter I shall explore some of the ethical aspects of communication and conclude with a consideration of some situations in which what counts as 'good communication' requires health professionals to make difficult moral judgements between competing ethical demands.

Medical educators have for many years argued for the importance of communication skills in good medical practice.

> Effective communication is essential to high-quality medicine; it improves patient satisfaction, recall, understanding, adherence and outcomes of care.
>
> (Silverman, Kurtz and Draper 1998a)

> Knowledge, communication skills, physical examination and problem solving are the four essential components of clinical competence that are the very essence of good clinical practice.
>
> (Silverman, Kurtz and Draper 1998b)

But what is *effective* communication? Browsing through a guide to effective communication for public speakers (or effective advertising) one might expect to find at least some of the following tips:

◆ Be well-prepared
◆ Speak clearly and accessibly (and entertainingly) in a language your audience understands.
◆ Know your audience, know who you are talking to. Empathize with them, listen to them and take note of their concerns.
◆ Get your message across. Be convincing in your arguments.

It is obvious from this fictional selection that effective communication, at least in a narrow sense, is insufficient by itself to guarantee the kind of 'good communication' required for good medical practice, even if some elements are indeed necessary. Very effective communicators can still be bad doctors and effective communication can be used for a very wide range of ends, both good and evil. This is made more obvious still when one considers who might count as exemplars of effective communication. A shortlist of paradigmatically effective communicators might include con artists, advertisers and dictators, each of whom is, for their success, as dependent upon the cultivation of excellent communication skills as any doctor. What this makes clear is that good medicine requires not simply *effective* communication but effective and *ethical* communication.

The aims of ethical communication

Perhaps the best way of getting at the difference between communication that is simply effective and that which is both effective and ethical, is to consider the range of ways, in addition to failures of effectiveness, in which communication in the consultation can go wrong. These might include:

- Failing to provide sufficient information for the patient to be able to make an informed choice about the available treatment options
- Coercing a patient into accepting, or rejecting, a particular course of action.
- Imposing treatment upon a patient irrespective of their wishes
- Not listening to the views and concerns of patients
- Deceiving patients, lying to them or not telling them the truth
- Being rude or unsympathetic towards patients
- Failing to treat patients in similar situations equally

What these examples of poor communication have in common is that they each exemplify different ways of failing to *respect patients as persons*. The importance in communication of relating to patients as persons is also emphasized strongly in the findings of the Kennedy Report.

> We are concerned here with attitudes—the frame of mind which the professional brings to the job. The pre-eminent attitude must be that the NHS is a service for the public. The needs of the patients must be the driving concern. This calls for a recognition of the need to establish and maintain good communication with patients and with fellow profession-als. It calls for a commitment to respect patients, and to be honest and open towards them. And here, honesty includes the obligation of professionals to be honest with themselves about their abilities. An attitude of public service also calls for the ability to convey uncer-tainty without fearing that it will appear weak. It calls for retaining and conveying a sense of open-mindedness in the dialogue which is the patient's journey. Perhaps most impor-tant of all, it calls for a sense of shared humanity, sympathy, understanding, an ability to engage with the patient on an emotional level, an ability to listen, an ability to assess how much patients wish to know about their condition and treatment, and an ability to convey information with clarity and sympathy. Caring is not just 'what nurses do'. It is what all healthcare professionals should do. In our view, therefore, the attitude of public service which we describe is the essence, the affirmation, of professionalism, not its antithesis.
>
> (Kennedy Report 2002a)

Respect for persons

But what would it mean to respect someone as a *person*? In his book The Value of Life, the philosopher John Harris argues that,

> The attitude to others that we call 'respect for persons' has two essential elements. They are essential in the sense that no one could coherently claim to respect others if their behaviour failed to exhibit both dimensions. Someone who has respect for person will show both,
> (1) concern for their welfare
> and
> (2) respect for their choices.
>
> (Harris 1985)

One can see immediately that these two components of respect for persons have their origins in the ethical theories described earlier. This makes the concept of respect for persons extremely useful in medical ethics, but it also suggests that the application of the concept will in practice be subject to the same tensions and conflicts. What are the implications of these two aspects of respect for persons for communication, and what should health professionals do when these two aspects come into conflict?

Ethical communication I: Respect for patient wishes

The second of Harris' principles, respect for the choices of persons, implies that ethical communication will be *patient-centred*. Patient-centred medicine with respect to this principle will be manifested in a genuine intention in the doctor to use communication skills in the consultation to achieve *valid* patient consent to (or refusal of) treatment options. That is, it will be concerned not only to respect patient choices per se but also to ensure that the decisions patients make in the consultation are, *informed, voluntary* and *competent.*

The implications for communication skills in the consultation are clear. For consent to (or refusal of) a treatment option to be informed, patients must have received sufficient information (in an accessible form), and had sufficient opportunity to ask questions and discuss options, and time to think, to enable them to make a genuinely informed decision. For patient choice to be voluntary, it must be made freely on the basis of their own wishes. The patient must be free from coercion either by the doctor, by other health professionals, by family members or from any other source e.g. financial or other inducements. The patient must be absolutely free to make choices other than the ones the doctor expects, or hopes for.

These two aspects of valid consent are mutually supportive. Two of the most common forms of coercion are the selective giving of information and deception. In the light of this relationship, the requirement that doctors place respect for patient choices at the heart of their communication requires a very high standard of openness and frankness with patients in the consultation. For, an implication of the argument that consent should be informed and uncoerced is that honesty and openness with patients are essential elements of effective and ethical communication. This is not unproblematic of course even in its own terms. Overloading patients with information can sometimes leave patients feeling disempowered and unable to make a decision. Despite this concern, it would appear to be a requirement of respect for persons that communication with patients should achieve a very high degree of truthfulness and involve the avoidance of all forms of deception. Some of the practical implications of this are that ethical and effective communication will:

- ◆ Involve breaking even very bad news compassionately and sensitively, but completely frankly.
- ◆ Not avoid the discussion of difficult decisions e.g. resuscitation, even where these are likely to be very distressing.
- ◆ Encourage discussion of the *real* reasons for difficult clinical decisions even where these are not entirely clinical e.g. resource allocation reasons for treatment refusal.
- ◆ Being honest and open about medical error and mistakes, whatever the legal or other implications.

I have suggested that valid consent should be informed and voluntary. In addition, consent to or refusal of treatment, to be valid, must be competently given. There will be many cases in medicine in which treatment decisions need to be made but where there is doubt about the patient's competence to make the decision. The key consideration in making such an assessment will be the question of the patient's competence *for this particular decision*. Patients may be incompetent in a range of areas of their life and yet competent to make a particular health care decision. It is of course particularly important not to assume that simply because a patient has a mental illness that they are incompetent to make any decisions about treatment. Despite this caveat there will clearly be some situations in which a treatment decision needs to be made about a patient who is incompetent. In such cases, respect for persons, in Harris' second sense comes to the fore. That is, concern for their welfare.

Ethical communication II: Concern for patient welfare

Harris argues that respect for persons involves both respect for their choices and also concern for their welfare. In cases where the patient is incompetent and there is no evidence of prior wishes (e.g. an advance statement) the relationship between these two principles is relatively straightforward. In such situations, there are no choices to be considered and doctors must act out of concern for their patients' welfare. That is, in their 'best interests'. In competent patients too, in general, these two concerns (choices and welfare) will be in harmony. Patients will usually want what is most likely to be of benefit to them. In such cases, respecting patient choices through the achievement of valid consent will satisfy both principles. In the vast majority of consultations grasping the demands of 'respect for persons' will be relatively straightforward and where practice does not in fact embody respect of this kind, it should be changed. As most doctors will know however, there are also occasions in which it is not clear what is required by 'respect for persons'. In such cases, where there is a conflict between patient wishes and the doctor's perception of patient welfare it is not always easy to assess what counts as ethical communication, or indeed, respect for persons.

Challenges to ethical communication

I have argued that ethical communication is patient-centred in a strong sense and will require high standards of openness and honesty combined with respect for the valid choices of patients made on the basis of such communication. But such an approach is not wholly unproblematic. There are at least four important situations in which patient-centredness, even with a competent patient, is challenged. These situations can be seen as posing questions both about the limits of respect for patient choice *and* about the limits of concern for patient welfare.

Patients who make the 'wrong' treatment choice

One situation in which the ethics of patient-centred medicine is challenged is where competent patients who have been provided with all the relevant information, in a supportive and effective consultation, make a treatment choice that the clinician feels is mistaken. An example might be a situation in which two treatment options are discussed for a life-threatening condition. One treatment option is much more effective than the other and much more likely to save the patient's life but comes with some significant but temporary side-effects. The other treatment has quite a low likelihood of saving the patient's life but has much milder side-effects. The patient chooses the second option because she 'doesn't like the sound of the side-effects'. In such a situation, to what extent is it legitimate for a clinician to 'encourage' or 'convince' the patient to see the merits of the other option? When does such 'encouragement' become unacceptable? The ethical question here is, how much convincing is compatible with respect for persons? The answer surely cannot be 'none' or 'never'. An alternative, and perhaps more uncomfortable way of putting the question for health professionals might be 'What are the limits of concern for patient welfare?'

Patients who make the 'wrong' moral choice

In other situations, patients may not be making poor treatment decisions but making judgements which the clinician feels are *morally* wrong. Consider a situation in which a patient is given a genetic test result which has implications for relatives, one of whom is currently pregnant and who might make more informed reproductive choices with this information. The patient refuses to share this information with his relative. If the seriousness of the harm caused to the relative is relatively small and does not meet the relevant standard or guideline for breaching confidentiality but the doctor does feel that the patient is making a morally wrong decision to keep this information from his relative, what should the doctor do? Is it acceptable for the doctor to initiate a discussion of the moral implications of the patient's choice? Or, does respect for patient choice and welfare mean that the doctor would be wrong to intervene? The question here again is, How much discussion of the moral implications and obligations of patient choices is compatible with respect for persons? Again, the answer must be surely not be 'none' or 'never'.

Patients who want no information at all

There are some patients who tell their doctor that they don't want any information at all about their illness or its proposed treatment. This puts the doctor concerned with effective and ethical communication in a difficult position. For her, all treatment decisions should be based on fully informed, voluntary patient choices. But what should she do when the patient's choice is to refuse involvement in the decision-making process? In such situations, whilst doctors will want to respect the patient's wishes not to be over-burdened with difficult and distressing information, they will want to ensure that the patient knows what treatment is planned and what the implications of this are for the patient. But does this conflict with patient-centredness where the patient has refused information? It does seem to. Nevertheless, this seems like a reasonable and acceptable thing for an ethical doctor to do. What are the limits of patient choice when it conflicts with the principle of 'respect for patient choice' itself?

Patients who refuse life-saving treatment

In situations where patients make informed, competent and voluntary decisions to refuse life-saving treatment the tensions between respect for patient choices and concern for their welfare reach their peak. In such situations we feel it appropriate to explore the patient's *reasons* for their choice, to make sure that they are competent and that the choice is informed and voluntary. Having satisfied ourselves that this is the case, such choices are currently respected. In the end we place respect for patient choice above concern for patient welfare. There might be several justifications for this. We might think that overall, placing great emphasis on patient choice brings about the greatest amount of patient welfare, even if in some individual cases, it does not. Alternatively we might think that competent patients are in the best position to make an assessment of what is in their own welfare. Or we might take the view, quite apart from concern about welfare, that we simply have an obligation to respect the informed and voluntary choices individuals make about their own lives, whatever we think about their relationship to the welfare of the chooser. On any of these models, the ethical choice to respect the choices of the patient will depend upon being reasonably certain that these are in fact the competent wishes of the patient, and that the patient has thought through the implications of their choice. This being the case, it will be the responsibility of the ethical doctor not simply to accept the choices and views of patients at face value but to challenge them when this is appropriate, in a supportive and constructive way. But what are the appropriate limits of such 'challenging'?

Conclusions

It is widely recognized that good communication skills are a necessary feature of good medical practice and that communication skills training is a core element of the training of good doctors. In this chapter I have argued that good communication in the consultation must be both effective and ethical and I have also argued that the measure of whether this is the case will in addition to its effectiveness, also be the extent to which it respects patients as persons. Respect for persons in this context means respecting the informed, voluntary choices of patients and being concerned with the promotion of their welfare. Each of these demands is justified in terms of the moral theories described earlier on in the chapter. In most cases, these two aspects of respect for persons will be in harmony. Both deontologists and utilitarians will agree. If adequately informed and supported patients will usually be concerned to make choices that are in their own best interests. There will however, be situations in which this is not the case. I have outlined four examples of such situations above. In situations such as these doctors will need to make judgements about the appropriate approach to communication. In such cases the required judgement will not simply be one about the most *effective* form of communication. The judgement required will be one between two or more moral principles. This will require moral judgement. For this, doctors will not only require training in the skills of effective communication but also complementary training and experience in moral judgement. This would seem to imply that effective communication skills training is only possible if it is taught in close collaboration with the teaching of ethics. Similarly, it can be seen from the above case scenarios, that any assessment of the ethical aspects of the consultation will need to pay particular attention to the modes of communication at work. Taken together, these facts would seem to call for a close relationship between, and perhaps even partial integration of, the teaching of ethics and communication skills to both medical students and qualified doctors. (Parker and Dickenson, 2001)

Finally, in this chapter I have for obvious reasons addressed the ethical and communication skills in the consultation from the perspective of the responsibilities of the doctor. I have not addressed the communicative responsibilities of patients themselves. Suffice to say, that communication to be effective, and ethical, must be engaged in genuinely and authentically from all sides.

> [T]here is a further dimension of equal importance [...]—what patients can do in the interview to influence communication and their own health care. Far from being passive recipients of changes that doctors adopt, patients have a major part to play in the process of the consultation. How individual patients can participate differently in the consultation, how they can take responsibility themselves to alter the doctor–patient relationship, how they can adopt a more active role in the interview are questions that deserve equal attention and investigation.
>
> (Silverman, Kurtz and Draper 1998c)

References

Beauchamp, T., Childress, J. (1994). *Principles of Biomedical Ethics*, 4th edition. Oxford: Oxford University Press.

Harris, J. (1985). *The Value of Life* p. 193. London: Routledge.

Kant, I. (2001 (1785)). *Groundwork of the Metaphysics of Morals* (Trans. Mary Gregor) Cambridge: Cambridge University Press.

Kennedy Report of the Bristol Inquiry, Kennedy Report (2002a). Accessed on 25th November 2002 at http://www.bristol-inquiry.org.uk/final%5Freport/report/sec2chap25_5.htm

Parker, M., Dickenson, D. (2001). *The Cambridge Medical Ethics Workbook*. Cambridge: Cambridge University Press.

Silverman, J., Kurtz, S., Draper, J. (1998a). *Skills for communicating with patients*, p. 1. Oxford: Radcliffe Medical Press.

Silverman, J., Kurtz, S., Draper, J. (1998b). *Skills for communicating with patients*, p. 1. Oxford: Radcliffe Medical Press.

Silverman, J., Kurtz, S., Draper, J. (1998c). *Skills for communicating with patients*, p. 3. Oxford: Radcliffe Medical Press.

Chapter 4

Overall plan of management of difficult conversations

Elisabeth Macdonald

Summary

This chapter summarizes a basic practical formula for the conduct of a first consultation and also, separately, for subsequent conversations.

Introduction

Let us now summarize a practical basic formula for many conversations between health professionals, patients and relatives. The shortlists in the boxes on this page will map your path through many conversations. However, it cannot be emphasized enough that each patient is individual and each circumstance different and unique to the situation. What is appropriate in one context may be far from appropriate in another. Use these checklists to create a constructive mind-set that will enable you to adapt to the situation in hand.

First consultations

First consultations

Meet with courtesy and frank approach—Smile!

Establish some personal contact

Explain time schedule

Solicit the patient's agenda in full. Try not to interrupt!

First consultations *(continued)*

Prioritize with patient agreement

Affirm empathy

Any other issues?

Focus on agreed priority issues

Construct with patient an agreed approach

Arrange next process (investigations, referral)

Any other issues?

Explore patient understanding

Arrange next appointment

1. *Meet with courtesy and frank approach.* When initiating a conversation with patients or relatives it is important to behave in a respectful, courteous and polite manner. Give your name and explain your position. Offer a handshake and seat the person comfortably.

2. *Establish personal contact.* It is helpful to start by establishing certain basic facts such as where they live, what they do, who are the important members of their friendship or family circle. This is a shorthand way of placing the individual patient in their personal context and offers reassurance that they as an individual are under consideration.

3. *Explain time schedule.* Explain what time is available and agree to prioritize.

4. *Solicit the patient's agenda and list of priorities.* Allow the patient to lead this part of the consultation. It will save you time later.

5. *Agree with the patient what are his or her principal concerns* and examine these in detail.

6. *Affirm your interest* in the issues mentioned and offer a sympathetic appraisal of them.

7. *Check again* that you are dealing with the main issues from the patient's point of view.

8. *Question closely* to elicit the information relevant to this issue. Cover all the topics of a 'standard' history, including the patient's own ideas, concepts and expectations.

9. *Formulate a plan* of action with the patient. Are investigations necessary? Should the patient be referred for a specialist opinion?

10. *Arrange appointments* in line with the agreed process.

11. *Check* whether any other issues are now ready to be volunteered.

12. *Arrange a convenient follow-up* appointment to discuss results, further thoughts, evolution of symptoms, etc.

Subsequent conversations

Subsequent conversations

Meet with courtesy and frank approach—Smile!

Establish some personal contact

Establish the patient's current knowledge

Repeat recent events to ensure that these are understood

Identify the next issues

Explain how the situation has developed or changed

Discuss the certainties, uncertainties, likely course of events and possibilities

Estimate the time frame

Ask what else the patient would like to know

Ask the patient to summarize

Give time for information to sink in

Arrange a further opportunity for discussion

1. *Meet with courtesy and frank approach* (see above).

2. *Establish some personal contact* (see above).

3. *Establish the patient's or relative's current knowledge of the situation.* It is pointless to pass on further, often complex, information without first establishing that previous information has been understood and digested. It is vital to check that the facts that have so far been established are clearly understood by the patient or family. Misunderstandings at this stage can lead the patient to misunderstand fundamentally the next piece of information that is offered.

4. *Identify the next issues.* Having established the background then identify the next issues to be covered. These may, for example, be the results of further tests. They may be the opinions given by other medical specialists or views that the patient and family have had an opportunity to clarify from their own end.

5. *Explain how the situation has developed or changed.* The new information may mean that a change in management strategy is required. It may, for example, imply that there is a problem that requires surgical intervention. On the other hand the new results may suggest a different form of medication or therapy. Alternatively, the picture may remain unclear and suggest that a further test may help to clarify the picture.

6. *Discuss the certainties, uncertainties, likely course of events and possibilities.* At this stage it is helpful to clarify what is certain about the situation. Often the associated uncertainties are much more numerous and need to be explained with care and

precision. Many lay people find the uncertainty, so often a part of medicine, the most difficult concept to follow. People feel that science and, in particular, medicine, is well researched and that facts should be both clear and explicable. The subtleties of different possible diagnoses and explanations for their condition are hard to conceive. It is then useful to discuss the most likely course of events given the current situation but also to mention the less likely possibilities. Medicine as we all know is full of surprises. Doctors need to explain with appropriate humility that they do not have all the answers and cannot predict the future in most circumstances.

7. *Estimate the time frame.* For most patients it is essential, and for many of paramount importance, to estimate the time frame for future events with a realistic range of possible eventualities. Disease can be notoriously variable in its severity, pace and evolution and many patients and their families need to know for practical purposes an outline of the best-case scenario as well as the worst.

8. *Ask what the patient would like to know.* At this stage it is useful to ask what else the patient would like to know or may not have fully understood. Often queries from previous conversations, which the patient has been mulling over at home surface at this point and reveal new voids in understanding that this conversation gives an opportunity to remedy.

9. *Patient summary.* Asking a patient to summarize the information in their own words helps them to register and digest the new information as well as giving an opportunity for corrections of misapprehension if appropriate.

10. *Give time for information to sink in.* New information is likely to take some time to sink in. If you have a moment to allow the patient to reflect it can allow them to articulate matters that would become a problem later.

11. *Next appointment.* When information of a complex or distressing nature has been imparted it is essential for the patient to know that a further opportunity is scheduled for the patient to discuss matters further.

Conclusions

This outline for conversations represents an ideal, which in busy medical practice cannot always be enacted. The absolute essentials are those of a frank and courteous approach to a clear relevant exchange of information between equal participants with an opportunity to follow up at a later date.

Chapter 5

The patient's perspective

Elisabeth Macdonald and Katherine Murphy

Summary

The Patients' Association, which represents one voice speaking for patients, summarizes a number of important problems seen from the patient's perspective. Health-care workers are also aware of many aspects of the doctor–patient interchange that are inherently problematic. Difficulties arise as a result of the subject matter of consultations as well as from the preconceptions, which patients bring to the exchange.

Views from the Patient's Association

From our point of view suggestions which would be beneficial to the patient are as follows—

In the hospital setting when a consultant is going to give bad news, it would be much kinder if he visited the patient on a 'one to one' basis without his entourage, and perhaps arrange for the nurse in charge to immediately go and chat with the patient after he leaves.

If a GP has received a report of bad news regarding one of his patients he should familiarise himself with the disease state and any relevant support groups before the patients appointment.

It would be helpful (or is this just a utopian ideal) if he could ring the patient and suggest they bring a companion to the appointment.

If any receptionist phones on behalf of the GP they must be specially trained when making a phone call of this kind. After a GP has given an adverse report to the patient perhaps he could suggest that they return a few days later for a further discussion of treatments/outcomes.

The patient is no longer the poor little person who sits in the corner with their arms tightly folded, knees crossed (typical defensive position) and listens to the doctor telling them what is going to be done to them. The patient is now supposed to be a partner, and not just someone that a doctor may do something to. The patient now works in conjunction with the doctor.

Patients are now well aware of the pressure of time on Doctors; they know that it is unlikely the Doctor will have enough time to explain a diagnosis properly and answer all the questions, it is important therefore that time is used constructively.

Patients increasingly want doctors to take account of their preferences and to involve them in choice of treatment and management of their condition. Many patients now want to play a part in their own care. They want doctors to help them to do this. Better communication between the doctor and the patient means that patients are less likely to accept a passive role as recipients of health care. Patients can be trusted to take more responsibility for themselves, especially when working with the whole clinical team across the whole range of services. By empowering individual patients they can each take more responsibility for their clinical condition.

Doctors still have a habit of using medical terminology that is unfamiliar to most patients. They are told they are suffering with Diagnosis X . . . . The patient has no idea what the Doctor is talking about, is sometimes not sure what part of the body is affected and unclear about the treatments offered. The explanation from Doctor to patient needs to be clear and simple and the Doctor must give the patient the opportunity to ask any questions.

Patients want to be more involved in their healthcare; this is not easy and takes far more imagination, consideration and doing things very differently. Patients today can get more information if they choose to fight their way through the many websites that exist. They may obtain more information than ever before if they consult the disease specific charities that fine-tune the data that exists. They may also gain information from the increasingly good medical journalism that now exists.

Katherine Murphy, Director of Communication, the Patient's Association
(20 November 2002)

Awareness of the patient's perspective

With these observations from the Patient's Association in mind what do practised doctors observe from their experience to be the factors that make conversations difficult from the patients' point of view?

Problems originate not only from the subject matter of consultations but also from the understandable anxiety with which the patient may approach the interchange.

Subject matter

Problems can arise from the subject matter of the conversation. The information received may contain bad news involving either a poor prognosis or a life-threatening illness. It may be that the patient has been dreading this conversation, fearing that it will confirm already worrying fears. They may be dreading confirmation of a serious diagnosis or of the reoccurrence of a serious illness. They may be worried about a poor prognosis or feel that their life is imminently under threat. Bad news on health issues adversely affects a person's view of their whole future.

Alternatively, the patient may be faced with burdensome news concerning lengthy or unpleasant treatment. The patient may understand that the treatment is necessary to improve quality of life or likelihood of survival but contemplation of the side-effects, discomfort, hospitalization and disruption of normal life can be profoundly intimidating.

Alternatively, they may receive frightening news about a condition for which no effective treatment is actually available. This may be unexpected news involving information that the patient has never had reason to contemplate. The conversation may contain an ugly surprise that had never before appeared on the patient's horizon. The patient is likely to be both factually and emotionally ill prepared for this kind of conversation.

Conversations involving genetic information may have implications not only for the patient, but also for the patient's relatives. Those affected may be parents, siblings, children and cousins as well as carers. The information may concern pre-programmed genetic disorders such as Huntingdon's chorea with grave implications for several family members and their dependants. Since the decoding of the human genome genetic information is becoming rapidly more relevant and available. For example, the identification of families predisposed to different forms of cancer may have profound implications in possible strategies for cancer prevention. The proper discussion of this sensitive and potentially damaging information requires skill and training and should only be delivered by well-prepared experts in the field of genetics.

Some conversations may concern current or future fertility. These discussions will therefore have implications for the patient's current or future relationships and can have profound psychological impact.

Some difficult conversations concern personal disfigurement and radical surgery. The necessity for major surgery such as mastectomy, prostatectomy or hysterectomy can be associated with deep emotional distress. There can be an actual or perceived affront to the patient's body image or personal identity. Disfigurement involving the amputation of an extremity or severe and socially obvious scarring can be extremely traumatic. The loss of a body part can give rise to grief for the loss of body image or function or both. Anxiety, depression and sexual problems are related to the magnitude and type of loss as well as the personal vulnerability of the patient (Maguire and Murray Parkes 1998). Adjustment may be necessary in planning for future living and earning. Loss of body image leads to loss of self-confidence and loss of some functions may have long-term effects on the patient's ability to keep afloat financially and support themselves and their family.

Some conditions carry with them a social stigma that patients find embarrassing or shameful. The diagnosis of venereal disease and, more recently, the social stigma surrounding the diagnosis of AIDS/HIV can raise acute anxiety and fear of rejection and isolation. In some circles, especially among the elderly and disadvantaged social groups, old-fashioned attitudes to diagnoses such as cancer or tuberculosis may lead to the patient being shunned by their community and this may be of grave concern to your older patient.

Discussions concerning the diagnosis of a psychological disorder or psychiatric illness can cause acute anxiety and distress. Psychiatric disease remains particularly poorly understood in our community and engenders fear and rejection among patients and relatives alike. Some senile illnesses such as Alzheimer's disease can point to future intellectual disintegration and loss of 'self' with, for some patients, terrifying prospects for themselves and their close relatives.

Patient problems over subject matter

1. Breaking bad news
2. News of unpleasant treatment
3. Frightening news when no treatment available
4. Unexpected news
5. News with genetic implications
6. News concerning fertility
7. Disfigurement
8. Social stigma
9. Psychological illness
10. Senile illness with loss of 'self'

Patient preconceptions

Patients may equally find conversations with doctors difficult because of problems arising from their anxiety-laden preconceptions. Patients may be hampered in their conversations with doctors by fear of the unknown. The truism that the worst fear is that of the unknown is as true in medicine as in the rest of life. Although fictional television series depicting life in hospitals and casualty departments have to a degree dispelled some myths about the closed environment in which health-care professionals work, they have equally created different myths and misconceptions. Some of these perceptions taken from the stereotypes of personalities and situations enacted on screen can complicate the patient's appreciation of staff and information. Casualty departments, for example, are in reality very different from the sensational, emotionally intense settings of television drama, and a serious diagnosis feels very different when the patient concerned is you yourself.

Patients may dread the consequences of the conversation at hand. These consequences may entail physical well-being, life expectancy, fear of pain or dying in pain. Patients may bring to this conversation the experiences of neighbours, friends or relatives who have had negative experiences and these may colour the patient's approach to their own health issues. The fear of dying in pain is particularly acute. Many patients confide that they know that everyone must die and they accept their own death but nevertheless dread the possibility of dying in pain.

Most people in society are remarkably ill informed about anatomical and medical terminology. The unfamiliar vocabulary entailed in medical discussions can be intimidating or poorly understood. The use of medical language and especially abbreviations, which are unintelligible to the patient, should be avoided. Simple diagrams can go a long way to dispel misapprehensions of this kind. It can be very helpful to draw a sketch of the part of the body involved with a simple representation of, for example, where a surgical scar will be or the position of a kidney or other abdominal organ. Give your sketch to the patient and it will serve as a reminder to the patient and also help answer the questions of relatives. For the same reasons many people welcome a written note of their diagnosis or the name of the treatment planned. This gives them the opportunity later to seek more information. Advice on appropriate and helpful websites is invaluable to the technically adept and wise counsel at this stage can prevent the patient wasting a lot of time surfing the net inappropriately. Well informed patients are more satisfied and less time consuming on the whole than those who are ill informed or widely misled by an inappropriate information source.

Patients are often fearful of appearing foolish or stupid when faced with information that they find hard to digest. There may be considerable embarrassment at their failure of understanding and a reluctance to reveal their ignorance and ask those questions that would clarify the issues involved. It is thoughtless and unhelpful to fall back on medical phraseology when talking to an individual who has no experience of this environment and its vocabulary.

Some problems in conversation arise from the patient's mistaken approach or incomplete understanding of their own situation. There is a great deal of relatively superficial medical information available in the lay press and patients may 'self-diagnose' in a way that leads them to have made faulty assumptions. As a result they bring to the consultation a closed mind and the potential for pursuing an entirely faulty approach to their situation. This may either overestimate or underestimate the seriousness of their condition. Patients' past experience of illness can also have a profound influence on their current situation. They may anticipate, for example, the same outcome as an unfortunate friend or relative some years ago with a similar but different condition. Lay perceptions of illness sometimes mean that patients have ideas about their illness or its treatment that are out of date or are at odds with current medical practice. This means that the health professional needs to correct the patient's misconceptions and dispel anxieties before progress can be made.

Patients may also fear a loss of privacy. Some clinical situations will require discussion of private matters that are normally kept to the patient themselves or at least within the family. These discussions may reveal secrets that the patient would very much prefer to remain hidden.

Some patients especially the elderly and the reticent can be intimidated by interaction with a forbidding person in a white coat. The label of 'doctor' and the status denoted by the white coat can cause some patients a loss of confidence that interferes with the free flow of information and explanation. Occasionally, the necessity to convey bad news stimulates transference of anger concerning the bad news to the doctor communicating it. This 'shoot the messenger' syndrome is one that doctors learn to accept and absorb in the short term as an understandable reaction to bad news. Fortunately, research has shown that it is only in circumstances when patients perceive their 'bad news' conversation in extremely negative terms that this transference is likely to persist (Barnett 2002). Doctors who communicate bad news in an unsympathetic, hurried and sketchy manner are understandably likely to attract anger and resentment tying together the 'bad' messenger with the 'bad' message.

Some patients have described their resentment at being 'managed by fear'. The diagnosis of some conditions, shall we say for example breast cancer, may require the discussion of a number of treatment options. There may be a whole sequence of necessary treatments such as chemotherapy, surgery, irradiation and hormone treatment, all of which need to be described in detail. All of these measures may involve side-effects and potential complications that need to be discussed. In explaining these treatments and the indications for each modality, the doctor will often try to put the problem in context by citing research work and statistics. These data can be extremely intimidating for the patient and create the impression for some patients that the doctor is 'coercing' the patient into receiving the whole series of treatments. Most people need time to digest this volume of information. Some patients, especially if they feel the consultation was hurried, feel that they are being manipulated by the fearful consequences of refusing treatment and hence being 'managed by fear'.

Patients thus bring to their medical consultations a wide variety of potential problems arising from the subject matter of the discussion or from anxiety-laden perceptions that colour the discussion. In order to achieve good quality communication all health-care professionals need to be aware of the kind of perceptions that patients may bring to the discussion. You need to be mindful of what you hear but equally it helps to be aware of what your patient is avoiding or is not saying.

Listen to your patient and to what the patient is not saying!

You need to do your best as Joseph Lister suggested to 'put yourself in a patient's place' and to imagine the impact of your words from the patient's point of view.

Patient perceptions that can hamper conversations

1. Fear of the unknown
2. Fear of consequences: loss of well being, life expectancy, dying in pain
3. Unfamiliar vocabulary
4. Fear of appearing foolish
5. Incomplete understanding, wrong approach
6. Fear of loss of privacy
7. Resentment at loss of control
8. Intimidation by 'white coat'
9. Resentment at being 'managed by fear'

Patient preparation for a consultation

What can patients or potential patients do to prepare ourselves for consultations with a doctor?

Lists

One commonly used strategy is to prepare ahead of time a list of the questions a patient would like to ask the doctor. This ensures that the patient has a personal checklist available that expresses his or her own list of priorities.

Several authors have investigated the efficacy of list-making as an aid to doctor–patient communication. One model involved the patient in handing in before the consultation a list of the topics he or she wanted to cover. This study found that when offered the opportunity to list important questions prior to an interview only about half of patients actually made use of this chance (Jones *et al.* 2002). This study, however, formed part of a larger randomized controlled trial of computer-based information and thus involved patients who were already quite familiar with talking to doctors. This observation may not therefore have been wholly typical. Some interesting points, however, did emerge. Fewer patients from socially deprived areas made use of lists and those patients who declined to list their questions cited the fact that they thought that doctors were too busy to read them or discuss them. One patient made the very sensible suggestion that he preferred to keep his list as a prompt rather than handing it in before the consultation. Doctors involved in this study felt that lists had been useful for about one-third of patients in raising queries that would not otherwise have been asked and felt that the small amount of time involved had been well spent.

Not all doctors view lists with enthusiasm, however. Middleton (1994) questioned primary-care trainers in Leicester and found that doctors' views of lists and the patients who bring them were ambivalent. Seventy-one per cent thought that they were an aid to clarifying problems but 67% also thought they would be time-consuming. Patients bringing lists were negatively described as 'heart-sink' or obsessional.

It would seem that the use of lists to clarify patients' queries, keep a consultation to the point and improve patient satisfaction has considerable potential, well worth further investigation, but that both parties, doctor and patient, need education in their best use.

Prompt sheets, coaching and workshops

Three other avenues have so far been reported in the search for ways to facilitate a patient's interview with a doctor. These are: the use of doctor-generated prompt sheets, coaching of patients in the art of asking questions and the organization of 'workshops' to prepare ill-equipped patients more thoroughly for an encounter with the doctor.

In one study, prompt sheets were prepared by medical staff anticipating the kind of concerns a patient might have and were provided before the consultation. These prompts were explained and endorsed by the doctors and worked through during the consultation. These proved to be a simple, inexpensive and effective means of promoting relevant patient questioning in the cancer consultation (Brown *et al.* 1999). Similarly, in the Netherlands, one group reported on the impact of a 'Frequently Asked Questions' checklist as a means of preparing coronary outpatients for a regular visit to their cardiologist (Martinali *et al.* 2001). Use of the checklist did not result in longer doctor–patient consultations, but did result in patients feeling less anxious before the visit and reporting positively on the usefulness of the checklist in preparing for a visit.

Barriers to communication

The increased difficulty experienced by ethnic minority groups in accessing health care has been frequently observed (Balarajan and Raleigh 1993). One new approach to this problem has been launched in the USA by a group based in Houston, Texas named 'EXCEED' (Excellence Centres to Eliminate Ethnic/Racial Disparities). By means of written information and workshops, this team of trainers or 'workshop co-ordinators' helps patients to recognize barriers to good doctor–patient communication, learn good patient communication techniques and practise the new skills (Ashton 1999).

Some of the barriers to good doctor–patient communication encountered by ethnic minority groups, but equally encountered by many patient groups and identified by this research are listed in the box.

Some barriers to communication experienced by ethnic minorities

- Language or cultural differences
- Limited access to health care
- Perception of inferior quality of care being offered
- Control by doctors of the conversation by an aggressive approach or medical jargon
- Stereotyping of cultural groups
- Time limits for clinic visits
- Excessive waiting times
- Age, gender
- Style of dress and grooming
- Wheelchair access

By means of a video presentation of one patient's adverse experience other patients are educated about the problems encountered and asked about similar situations experienced personally or by family and friends.

On the other hand this workshop also looks at those communication skills that should be expected from a doctor. The setting is that of a community in the USA but the principles apply world-wide.

The following checklist is offered at the workshop. Your doctor should . . .

1. Introduce himself/herself.

2. Ask you to describe your problem.

3. Give information on your condition and tests.

4. Provide a diagnosis.

5. Give instructions for treating your condition.

6. Explain things in a manner you can understand.

7. Know the latest medical advances.

8. Take time to answer questions.

9. Listen to you.

10. Display positive feelings toward patient and family.

11. Show his/her understanding of your situation.

12. Express himself or herself.

13. Maintain confidentiality about information you provide.

14. Offer language translation or assistance if appropriate.

15. Return your phone calls in a reasonable amount of time.

16. Encourage you to participate.

This workshop also prepares patients by listing some useful tips to improve technique in the consultation:

1. Prepare for your doctor's visit by setting goals. Write down problems. Share information with your doctor.

2. Take notes during the doctor's visit. Think about what you really want to say. Focus on one point at a time.

3. Ask questions.

4. Be assertive. Express your health concerns and explain any important cultural or religious beliefs.

This particular workshop then goes on to use some simple clinical conditions to enable the participants to practise their consultation skills and finally gives the patients a written reminder checklist to help them at their next visit to the doctor.

This kind of initiative is time consuming but may have a role in some of the more underprivileged areas of our society to bolster the self-confidence of people who otherwise find the medical environment profoundly intimidating.

References

Ashton, C. (1999). *Journal of the American Medical Association*, **282** (No. 24), 2422 (JAMA Patient Page).

Balarajan, R., Raleigh, V.S. (1993). *Ethnicity and Health: a guide for the NHS*. London: Department of Health.

Barnett, M. (2002). Effect of breaking bad news on patients' perceptions of doctors'. *Journal of The Royal Society of Medicine*, **95**, 343–7.

Brown, J., Butow, P.N., Boyer, M.J., Tattersall, M.H. (1999). Promoting patient participation in the cancer consultation: evaluation of a prompt sheet and coaching in question asking. *British Journal of Cancer*, **80**(1–2), 242–8.

Jones, R., Pearson, J., McGregor, S., Barrett, A., Harper Gilmour, W., Atkinson, J.M., Cawsey, A.J., McEwen, J. (2002). Does writing a list help cancer patients ask relevant questions? *Patient Education and Counselling*, **47**, 369–71.

Maguire, P., Murray Parkes, C. (1998). Coping with loss: surgery and loss of body parts. *British Medical Journal*, **316**, 1086–8.

Martinali, J., Bolman, C., Brug, J., van den Borne, B., Bar, F. (2001). A checklist to improve patient education in a cardiology outpatient setting. *Patient Education and Counseling*, **42**(3), 231–8.

Middleton, J. (1994). Written lists in the consultation: attitudes of general practitioners to lists and the patients who bring them. *British Journal of General Practice*, **44**(384), 309–10.

Chapter 6

The doctor's perspective

Elisabeth Macdonald

Summary

Doctors in consultation are normally reluctant to cause distress and hesitate to antagonize patients. They may well be fearful of their own inability to explain or to answer questions clearly and worried about making mistakes and getting things wrong. In specific clinical circumstances doctors need to prepare for very special aspects of difficult conversations. Issues emerging at the end of life concerning medical care and its modification, and many types of 'bad news' conversations are discussed. The effective communication of clinical risk and the disclosure of errors offer a particular challenge.

General perceptions

As we progress through medical training and early clinical experience, doctors are exposed to a wide variety of clinical environments and specialities. Along this path each of us makes a decision about which aspect of medical practice attracts us most. It is interesting to speculate on the factors that influence these decisions. I would suggest that an important part of this decision relates to the doctor–patient relationship. Some of us may be attracted by the purely scientific and intellectual aspects of medicine and prefer to work in a pathology department or diagnostic X-ray unit. In these circumstances personal exposure to patients and communication with families can be minimal. In contrast, specialities such as psychiatry, dermatology and oncology depend heavily on communication skills to practise effectively by combining intellectual discipline with the personal application of science. Our choice of career probably reflects not only our personality but also our perceived facility with communication and personal interaction. Some of us have an easy open manner and can talk to anyone. Others are more reticent, growing up in families that are more reserved, less extrovert and less expressive.

Whatever our background many doctors are reluctant and even fearful to engage with patients. First, there is reluctance to cause distress. Doctors are aware that patients are often anxious and frightened, dreading the very news that the doctor seeks to communicate. Good health is an essential commodity upon which the quality of all our lives depends. Sad news about health can cause great distress, not only to the patient but also their relatives and carers. Doctors seek to minimize distress and if poorly trained in delivering adverse information may seek to avoid the main issues or to vacillate and obfuscate in the hope that the patient will not realize the full meaning of the doctor's words. This potentially leaves the patient feeling confused, depressed and sometimes angry. Good communicators on the other hand become skilled at breaking bad news gently, in a realistic but sympathetic way that is carefully graded and timed. It is unfair on the patient to conceal unpleasant facts but reality does not mean brutality. It is possible to minimize the patient's distress by as it were taking your place alongside them, sympathizing with their predicament, negotiating an agreed policy and assisting the patient to achieve the best possible outcome in the circumstances.

Honesty does not mean brutality

Inexperienced doctors are often fearful of their inability to explain clearly what a diagnosis means and to explain its implications. They may feel inadequately prepared to answer questions and to provide the depth and scope of information that the patient requires. In these circumstances it is perfectly acceptable simply to say that you do not know but that you will ask your senior colleagues and come back to the patient with the information or arrange for the patient to be seen by a more experienced colleague in the near future.

Doctors are often fearful of being wrong. There seems in our culture to be an expectation that doctors always know the answers. In the complex world of modern medicine it is not unusual for doctors to reach a preliminary conclusion that is flawed or later contradicted. This can cause a crisis of self-confidence for the doctor as well as a loss of trust on the part of the patient. Although uncertainty is hard to live with, it is wiser to suggest a range of possibilities than to hazard a guess and be wrong.

When talking to patients, doctors are often reluctant to antagonize them and their relatives especially over sensitive issues such as those touching on personal or sexual relationships. Even when there are good clinical indications for seeking this information doctors may feel uncomfortable 'prying' into areas normally reserved for the family alone. Seams of family guilt, tension or strife may be unearthed, which, if insensitively handled, can antagonize the family and lead to a breakdown in goodwill and cooperation. Family members do not necessarily share attitudes to important issues especially across generations and it is wise not to assume that all (or any!) family functions harmoniously with goodwill on all sides. Opposing views may be exposed within a family over such matters as the wisdom of a risky operation and strain uneasy relationships. Discussion of an unexpectedly bad prognosis can engender ill feelings relating to both emotional and financial areas of concern and in certain circumstances even the revelation of a surprisingly good prognosis can raise new problems for the future. Who will assume the responsibility of caring, for example, for an elderly relative, where will they be nursed and for how long? What will happen to the family home?

Doctors being merely people have a natural desire to avoid provoking anger, annoyance or adverse reactions. Even when doctors are gentle, diplomatic and sympathetic some patients and their families will react with anger directed at the doctor. It is not surprising that faced with the patient whose attitude is angry, the doctor feels reluctant to expose him or herself to the unpleasant experience of being on the receiving end. In extreme circumstances some demanding families go so far as to threaten harm to medical and nursing staff and fear of physical harm in certain circumstances is a genuine concern for doctors. We live in a society where violence and threatening behaviour are common currency and antisocial individuals can be patients too. The management of communication with difficult personality styles and strong emotions is dealt with in the next chapter.

Problems for doctors

1. Reluctance to cause distress
2. Fear of inability to explain and answer questions
3. Fear of contradiction or being wrong
4. Reluctance to antagonize
5. Fear of patient's anger, annoyance or adverse reaction
6. Fear of physical harm

The practice of any form of medicine requires constructive interaction with patients, relatives and colleagues. There are, however, in addition certain specialties in which very special well thought out levels of communication are particularly important. Some of these special circumstances are described in the following pages.

Special circumstances

1. Intensive care: discussions concerning cardiopulmonary resuscitation
2. Intensive care: withdrawal of life support
3. Organ donation
4. Withdrawal of active treatment
5. The dying patient
6. Advance directives or 'living wills'
7. Breaking bad news
8. Breaking news of unexpected death
9. Multiple bad news
10. Breaking bad news of uncertain prognosis
11. Discussion of medical risks
12. Disclosure of errors

Special circumstances

The patient in intensive care: including discussions concerning cardiopulmonary resuscitation (CPR)

The clinical context

Although the indications for CPR are frequently discussed between medical and nursing staff in order to clarify the proposed management of individual cases, discussion with the patient himself or herself is more problematic. It is important from the outset to be aware that there is no simple 'prescription' as to how to conduct these conversations. Each patient's situation is unique and there is no 'one way' that is appropriate in all circumstances. These discussions are often regarded with trepidation by junior medical staff. This reticence probably stems from a perception that the patient is already physically unwell, emotionally stressed, and from both these points of view therefore particularly psychologically vulnerable.

Intensive care of patients in a specialized unit can raise a wide variety of issues and CPR represents one of a number of possible treatment options. CPR is clinically indicated in the event of cardiac arrest. It is important to differentiate to begin with that there are two separate causes of cardiac arrest: those that arise from disease of the heart itself, usually the result of coronary artery blockage, and those that result from severe disease of other organs, such as renal failure.

Primary cardiac arrest occurs usually as a result of a heart attack when the sudden loss of blood supply to part of the heart triggers a lethal disturbance of cardiac rhythm. If CPR is applied immediately then there is a very high chance that the patient will survive. This was the basis on which coronary care units and paramedical training have been developed to treat patients with heart attack. The main risks of

CPR to the cardiac patient who is successfully resuscitated are those of pain from broken ribs and cerebral damage. Brain damage can be permanent due to the lack of adequate blood supply to the brain before resuscitation was effectively achieved.

The second form of cardiac arrest is secondary to some other non-heart problem that leads, for example, to biochemical disturbance causing secondary cardiac arrest. The results of CPR for secondary cardiac arrest are very poor indeed. Virtually all patients die but occasionally some survive. Those patients who survive reportedly almost never leave hospital. This group of patients are already suffering from an advanced illness and in this case the principal risk is that CPR may be successful and the patient will be kept alive only to carry on suffering from their advanced illness in a prolonged dying process. Many patients will opt not to undergo CPR in this condition but there are patients, especially young patients or those with young families who choose to have anything possible done to keep them alive. It is unacceptable to some religious groups ever to 'give up' if there is any chance of survival (see Chapter 12).

For patients with advanced illness the issue of CPR is just one of many treatment options that could prolong life. Other options available in the intensive care unit such as artificial respiration, renal dialysis, parenteral nutrition, antibiotics or blood transfusion represent treatment options also needing joint decision making.

In this context it is more helpful to open a conversation about CPR with a more general discussion asking how the patient feels things are going, what he or she is most worried about in the future, and checking what issues about 'active' treatment the patient has considered. One can then move into questions about specific treatment, including CPR.

Guidelines on CPR

Guidelines for the conduct of decision making about CPR were drawn up in 1999 by the British Medical Association, The Royal College of Nursing and the UK Resuscitation Counsel in consultation together.

All patients in hospital should be considered eligible for CPR. However, these guidelines state that it is appropriate to consider a 'do not resuscitate' (DNR) decision in the following circumstances:

1. CPR is unlikely to be successful ('futile'). In other words there is a fundamental medical cause preventing success (e.g. ventricular rupture).

2. CPR is not in accord with the recorded, sustained wishes of the patient who is mentally competent.

3. Where CPR is not in accord with a valid advanced directive (living will).

4. Resuscitation is likely to be followed by a length and quality of life that would not be in his best interest for the patient to sustain.

When appropriate these factors should be discussed sensitively with the patient and their family.

The process of decision making

(Ethox: University of Oxford 2000)

1. If it is decided that resuscitation would be futile for sound medical reasons then a Do Not Resuscitate (DNR) order can be recorded.

2. If resuscitation is not judged to be clinically futile it is then necessary to assess the patient's competence to take part in a discussion concerning CPR. The assessment of a patient's 'competence' or 'capacity' to make effective judgements on his or her own behalf is of fundamental importance to the practice of good medical care. Clear guidelines are widely available and it is the duty of all health-care professionals to be well versed in both the ethical principles and the practical requirements. (See for example the GMC booklet 'Seeking patients' consent: the ethical considerations'.)

3. If the patient is not thought competent to take part in decision making or does not wish to discuss the issue then the doctor should consider discussing the issue with the patient's family in order to help make a judgement. No one can either consent to or refuse treatment on the part of any other adult individual but it is none the less wise to seek the opinion of family members who can reflect the patient's previous attitudes. If the length and quality of life after resuscitation could be worthwhile for this patient then a DNR order should not be made. However, if the length and quality of life after resuscitation is likely to be unbearable and judged to be worse than death itself then a DNR order is reasonable.

4. When a patient is competent to hold such a discussion then the issues should be explored with the patient. If the patient completely refuses resuscitation when considering hypothetical cardiopulmonary arrest then the DNR order is properly recorded. If the patient would like a resuscitation attempt then no DNR order is given.

Legal considerations in the involvement of family members

(Ethox: University of Oxford 2000)

The legal position with regard to do not resuscitate 'orders' follows from the process summarized above and in the light of the law on consent. The key points are:

1. Resuscitation is to be regarded as a treatment like any other.

2. If the patient is incompetent to discuss the issue, the doctor must weigh up the situation on his behalf with appropriate advice and treat in the patient's best interest.

3. The patient's best interests may be served by withholding resuscitation.

4. A doctor is not obliged to provide futile treatment even at the patient's request.

5. A competent adult patient can refuse resuscitation (or any other treatment offered).

6. No one can give or withhold consent for resuscitation on behalf of an incompetent adult patient. In particular family members can neither refuse nor demand such treatment. Good medical practice, however, dictates that the family should be involved in these discussions in order to maintain confidence and communication and to clarify if necessary the patient's likely wishes in the light of previous family discussion.

Families often have strong feelings on the matter of resuscitation both in favour and against and these need to be carefully explored. Some families may feel that their loved ones have been subjected to enough distress, discomfort, pain and indignity as a result both of their disease and its treatment and that to subject them to further unpleasant measures with little likelihood of success is simply to add insult to injury.

On the other hand there are families that seek to prolong the life of a loved one by any means available. Some cultures regard 'giving up' as contrary to their religious faith and can demand that all measures, including CPR are undertaken no matter how unlikely is the chance of success. Exploring and clarifying these views in a sensitive manner can prevent misunderstanding and antagonism in the event of later cardiac arrest.

Unless a patient specifically asks it is probably unhelpful to describe the process of CPR in detail. The patient is unconscious at the time and unaware of the process. The details of the resuscitation process can seem very frightening and it is important not to intimidate or appear to 'bully' patients into agreeing a DNR decision, which should concern the principle rather than the process.

In discussing something as emotive and complex as CPR we also all need to avoid creating a situation in which we may seem to be justifying our own decision by seeking 'informed consent'. The risk is that the patient is not actually truly involved and is not given real choice but feels compelled to agree with the doctor.

If a doctor opens a discussion about CPR, perhaps on a negative note, it is important to be prepared for the fact that the patient may not agree that resuscitation should not be attempted and where the patient is competent and the attempt is not regarded as 'futile' then the patient has every right to opt for resuscitation.

One example of a discussion concerning CPR will be found in the second section of this book (Appendix I).

Intensive care: withdrawing life support

Intensive care units offer life support in a variety of life-threatening situations. Many units are attached to large casualty departments but there are also more specialized units whose patients are transferred from operating theatres or who work closely with units specializing in, for example, neurosurgical or neurological disorders, coronary care or liver disease.

Communication with the patient may be prevented by the patient's clinical condition and it is often attention to the family's understanding that is the chief communication challenge for the health-care team.

The clinical context

The majority of patients are admitted to these specialist units from hospital wards where their condition has been observed to be deteriorating. After a variable period of intensive therapy patients will either improve or fail to improve irrespective of the fact that they are maintained on life support systems. At some point it may be necessary for the health-care team to reach the decision that further treatment has no hope of reversing the patient's deterioration and that further attempts to keep the patient alive are futile. It may be necessary therefore for the health-care team to decide that active treatment and life support should be discontinued. The evolution of this decision and the process of treatment discontinuation form the basis of the conversations between doctors and members of the patient's family. It is usually the role of the consultant staff to take a lead in these discussions and each consultant will handle the conversation in their own way with slight differences in style, personal nuances and personal interpretation.

The decisions on discontinuation of treatment are those of the multidisciplinary health-care team. The family in the UK is normally excluded from the actual decision making for three main reasons. First, the patient's medical condition is the primary reason for the decision taken and this is not something with which the family is familiar. Secondly, families are not, in law, in a position to accept or refuse treatment on the part of another adult person. Thirdly, the burden of responsibility for discontinuation of treatment can weigh heavily in the form of guilt on those family members who do participate in such a decision and this is best avoided.

Early stages of communication

When patients are first admitted to this kind of unit the first messages to the family tend to be those of 'doom and gloom'. It is felt that it is in fact wiser and ultimately kinder to prepare relatives for the worst. Any less bad news then seems less painful. If on the contrary the relatives' hopes are raised initially but in fact an adverse outcome ensues then this is doubly hard to accept. Families are rarely given more than a 50% estimate of chance of their relatives surviving. It will be explained at the outset that the team is doing all that can be done with optimal drugs, support, antibiotics, renal dialysis, etc. and that this will continue as long as is necessary for the benefit of the patient.

In the first conversation the doctors may explain that theirs is a 'very honest unit'. They will explain from the start that they will not hide any information from the family concerning their relative. In view of the fact that the patient is already in the intensive care unit doctors do not usually feel it helpful at this stage to enquire whether the patient has expressed views about intensive care units and intensive therapy in their earlier life unless the family raises these issues.

Doctors stress the importance of setting the stage when the patient is first admitted to the unit. They ask the family in detail what they know and understand about their relative's illness. Nursing staff will also take this opportunity to refer back to the data established on admission of the patient to the hospital and clarify potentially important and sensitive information concerning issues such as religion and next of kin. It is vital at this early stage to ask the family to give clear guidance about the issues surrounding death and the rituals observed in the event of death, which are of significance to them as a family. Severe distress at a later date can inadvertently be caused if the team is unaware of the procedures that a family would like observed (see below and also Chapter 12).

Families will also find it reassuring when the care team assures them that someone will always come and find them if things are going wrong. Many units work on the basis that if all is proceeding as planned there is less need to keep the relatives up to date with the minutiae of care. They will not necessarily speak so often if all is going well. On the other hand if problems are developing the team will try to ensure that the family is on hand and kept fully informed.

Later stages of communication: the process of withdrawal of life support

After a period of time on maximal therapy there may come a stage when further escalation of treatment is not possibly beneficial to the patient. In this situation further 'treatment' would simply be regarded as prolongation of the dying process and this needs to be sensitively explained to families. It is explained that there is no hope of increasing the patient's survival and that to continue invasive procedures is simply prolonging the patient's existence in limbo and postponing their inevitable death. Further treatment in these circumstances would be futile. The exact format of this conversation will depend heavily on the team's relationship with the family. If a patient has only recently (perhaps over the last 12 hours) been admitted to the unit then the patient's supportive care will be maintained while the family adjusts to the situation and rapport is established with the health-care team. If the patient has been in the unit for several weeks then the team will be more immediately explicit once the point of futility has been reached.

Summary of the procedure

The aim of withdrawing life support when death is expected is to remove treatments that are no longer indicated and do not provide comfort for the patient. Doctors in this type of unit do not withdraw treatment for comfort. This process seeks to reduce as far as is possible the level of distress both for the patient and their family. The only rationale for tapering life-sustaining treatment is to allow time to control the patient's symptoms. Patients are sedated during the process as treatment would be potentially unpleasant if they were awake. Analgesia in combination with sedation is maintained. As it is also felt that severe thirst can be unbearable this is avoided by nasogastric feeding. An explicit plan is drawn up for the withdrawal of support and the handling of complications should they arise. This is discussed in detail with relatives and time given for the family to absorb this information. Most families are unaware that the majority of deaths occurring in intensive care units happen after withdrawal of support and this can be reassuring to relatives. In order to keep the patient comfortable they are sedated to a baseline where they will not respond to painful stimuli. The medication has both amnesic and euphoric effects. Those patients who have eventually recovered have described their only memories of this period as being those of family voices talking around them and of rubbish bins clanging shut!

Where support involves, as it often does, the use of artificial ventilation analgesia is increased to cover any current and anticipated levels of physical pain. Mechanical ventilation is one of the few life support treatments that often cannot be stopped abruptly. The common approach to stopping ventilation is gradually to reduce the fractional inspired oxygen concentration to that of room air while reducing ventilatory support to zero with appropriate dosing of narcotic cover. The transition from full ventilatory support to extubation or humidified air usually takes from 15 to 30 minutes. Families should, however, be warned that death, although expected, is not certain and timing may vary.

When a decision is taken to discontinue treatment the doctors and nurses work closely with the family. Alarm mechanisms are switched off and family wishes followed as far as is possible. Occasionally, for example, beds are pushed together so that families can be in close physical contact with their dying relative.

One of the drawbacks of a busy intensive unit is the lack of privacy .The noisy hilarity of the day-to-day life of the unit continues around the dying patient. Some feel that this may not be appropriate at the end stages of life. However, many families appreciate being included in the life of the unit and value the reassurance of the fact that life is carrying on normally around them.

It is not unusual for family strife to be exposed at such stressful times. In some parts of the world family assent (as opposed to consent) is required before discontinuing active therapy. This is not the legal situation in the UK. If family dynamics are contentious then staff will try to involve everyone in decision making and to be as inclusive as possible.

The basis of communication between family and staff is that of trust. Anger is not commonly seen but may, rather surprisingly, surface when the family has been warned that a patient will die and in fact the patient lives longer than expected. Families don't cope well with doctors' inability to forecast the timing of death. Often the team will explain in the early stages that they are actively treating the patient for a small chance of success and that 'futility' has not yet been achieved. This is a difficult concept for relatives to grasp focused as they are on their fear of death.

From the staff point of view it is most difficult to take the family through a dying process when the patient has been well aware of their situation on admission. Conversations with the family are particularly difficult and distressing in such circumstances.

> I perceive communication with the family as a pivotal area of my job. The delivering of bad news and communication with families is as important to me as caring well for the patient.
>
> The most difficult problems for us as medical staff to deal with are those patients who come in and become very sick very fast. There is no opportunity to establish rapport either with the patient or the family. Most difficult are those patients who come in severely acidotic who are alert, talking and very scared.
>
> Liver Unit Intensive Care Consultant (Dr Julia Wendon The Liver Unit, Kings College Hospital, London, Personal communication)

Management of differences of opinion and strong emotions

When families are angry it is important to sit down and listen in order to defuse the anger. Anger should be confronted not with anger but with recognition and enquiry. It is often important to allay unfounded suspicions that in another previous hospital or unit something inappropriate has been done. Blame is usually neither correct nor worthwhile and the relatives' energy is better conserved to support each other. A clinical psychology unit can provide considerable help here. Silence can be very useful followed by, for example, 'Is there anything you want to ask me?'

Another difficulty can arise when there are multiple consultants involved in the care of one patient. It is sometimes necessary to request colleagues not to be 'upbeat' in talking to the family. Most intensivists see their main role here as that of a diplomat. Often surgeons or other physicians closely involved with previous care have a vested interested in their patient and it is sometimes necessary to allow these clinicians 'a grieving process' as well as the family. Different levels of care lead to different involvement. It is important always to give the patient the benefit of the doubt and to carry on longer rather than with less time and patience.

Some families simply don't like the person of the doctor. In these circumstances a good working relationship is difficult to establish with the family and it is wise to get a colleague to talk to them. Part of the intensive care doctor's role is to make the patient's death as comfortable as possible for the relatives as well as the patient.

It is essential always to return to the subject of the patient and to ensure and then to stress that the patient is not suffering. When managing the end of a patient's life it is important to be consistent, especially in discussion of the role of analgesia and sedation. In the case of patients who are severely brain damaged or are brain dead there will not be, by definition, any awareness or sensation and therefore for the patient no suffering. It is important to be clear with the family that the patient is not suffering and it is for this reason that they will not need analgesia and sedation.

Doctors seek to stress the dignity of the patient and that it is undignified to carry on giving unnecessary treatment. Sometimes it is helpful to sit down and say something like, 'Can we imagine what your husband/father would say if he were here? Would he want to carry on in these circumstances?' (with a drip, nasogastric tubes, ventilator, etc.). Quite often the family will volunteer the view that 'No, he wouldn't like that' and this can help the relatives reconcile themselves to the reality of the patient dying.

In appropriate circumstances it may be sensible to encourage children to visit the ITU. Children are remarkably resilient and parents may need to be encouraged in the decision to involve children. This can prevent later regret on the part of both parents and children that they were not involved at the end or failed to pay their last respects and say 'Goodbye'.

Occasionally within the multidisciplinary team there may be differences of opinion about the management of the patient. Discussion is centred on resolving these differences and takes place in a multidisciplinary open ward round, in which the whole team participates. Conflict can be constructive, uncovering differences in values and legitimate concerns that have been inadequately discussed. Improved communication about goals and treatment options will successfully resolve most conflicts. Consultants usually have an open door policy and are open to discussion with family or team members at any stage. Occasionally, young nurses feel that patients are being 'tortured' by their treatment. It is helpful to explain that the patient 'will want to survive' if this is possible and hence will find the treatment acceptable.

It is also important to prevent families splitting the team. If, for example, one doctor is described as taking a different approach then another may reply, 'Yes, that is exactly what I am saying in a different way'.

Some relatives appear to seek out apparent differences of approach or emphasis to create divisions and it is wise for a team to be consistent and not defensive about differences.

Cultural differences

Do not underestimate the intelligence of other ethnic groups who may not have received a great deal of formal education but can none the less be very astute and can learn very quickly. On occasions the apparently well-educated family on the other hand can entirely miss the point. It is often only when such a family begins to ask questions that this reveals how little they have in fact understood.

Some families remain at odds with the realistic expectation of the health-care team. Such families are unable to come to terms with an impending death even when the health-care team has been explicit in explaining that the outlook is very poor. Some families still end such a conversation with 'So when will he be coming home?'

This form of denial may be either submissive or aggressive. Often there is an ethnic or cultural background to these differences of approach. Some cultures believe that doctors are irrelevant and that God will decide. In some ways this can be easier for the doctor as if a patient dies this can be seen as God's will. On the other hand it can be difficult when families require the doctor to carry on with active treatment when clinically this is not felt to be appropriate. One way to handle this is to ask the family what they themselves understand to be the situation. If the family is able to articulate for themselves the fact that they know the situation is very serious this may enable them to move on to a more realistic understanding. It can be very helpful for a member of the nursing staff from the same community to spend time with the family to explain the approach of the health-care team. (See also Chapter 12 for a fuller discussion of cross-cultural issues.)

Otherwise, cultural differences do not feature largely in the ITU. It can appear, however, to be a disaster for some families if death occurs after 3 p.m. on a Friday for the patient whose religion requires them to be buried within 24 hours. Death certificates are not available on Friday nights and over the weekends. It is necessary to explain to the family that these technicalities are beyond the hands of the medical staff. Among many minority ethnic communities most conversations are conducted with male members of the family and there can be some concern about what support is being given to the female members of the family.

Post-mortem requests

Referrals to the coroner can be regarded as extremely stressful to many families. It is very difficult for them to accept that their loved one is in a sense the 'property of the coroner'. The public have recently become antagonistic to post-mortem examinations and even to simple post-mortem biopsy. Very limited post-mortem investigations can be very informative and useful. It can, for example, be very helpful in liver disease to obtain a very small liver biopsy, simply a true cut needle biopsy, to establish the underlying pathology leading to death and families can be comforted when this reveals the diagnosis from which their loved one died. It can be very difficult for families if doctors are unable to tell them with certainty the cause of death. For instance, most acute liver disease is associated in the public mind with self-harm and alcohol abuse and in conditions where this is not the case families find it very stressful if they are unable to 'claim' a diagnosis.

If a Coroner's post mortem is required take the family carefully through the rules and explain why they exist. These rules were framed for the benefit of the whole society. In these situations poorly communicating doctors are those who manifestly fail to be at one with the family. They as it were 'keep their starched white coat on'. Good communication involves explaining in a systematic and honest way.

Role of the general practitioner

It can be extremely helpful when important decisions are to be made concerning discontinuation of treatment to contact the general practitioner (GP). Many good GPs know their patients well and can give useful insight into the patient's past attitude to the role of intensive care. The patient may have prepared an advanced directive or previous discussions with the GP amounting to a verbal advanced directive may clarify the patient's attitude.

Failure to inform the GP of a patient's death can put the GP in a very difficult position in relation to the family with an inappropriate response to the grieving family in ignorance of the fact that the patient has died. This failure to inform the GP practice can lead to antipathy between primary care and the intensive care unit.

Maintaining balance in intensive care work

Junior staff may worry that they will become overinvolved emotionally with their patients. Although professionalism helps to protect against this it is probably inevitable that some degree of overinvolvement ensnares the tired and caring doctor once or twice a year, and there are those who argue that if it doesn't you are probably in the wrong job!

In order to maintain equilibrium and survive emotionally oneself in this kind of work it is important to feel secure in ones own clinical skills and confident that it is despite and not because of your best care and that of your team that the patient has lost their life. The death has occurred despite your care and not as a result of it. To keep these issues in perspective it is helpful to vary the work pressures if possible; for example, alternating periods of frontline clinical work with research in rotating weeks. It is important to take adequate time out from frontline medicine. It is also important to have the right personality for the job, sympathetic but strong-minded, and an inspirational teacher often inspires such doctors to emulate their 'boss' and choose this speciality. (See also chapter below on Maintaining balance.)

Many intensive care doctors believe in actively debriefing the team together in a relaxed and convivial atmosphere, often in the pub after work. Many feel this is the best way of reducing stress levels and more effective than formal counselling. Many in this line of work do not believe that counselling is helpful in that it creates a feeling of dependency and need to talk rather than developing coping skills. Needless to say opinions differ.

Organ donation

It is now regarded as the duty of an intensive care unit doctor to seek organ donation when this is feasible and appropriate. The first essential for the doctor, however, is to deal with all aspects of an individual patient's death. The doctor can only then turn with a clear conscience to the question of organ donation. Organ transplantation is now so successful, the benefits so clearly defined and the shortage of organs so acute that a positive approach is amply justified in social terms (C. Rudge, Medical Director UK Transplant, personal communication, 2003).

In the past intensive care specialists have felt that there was a conflict of interest between their duty to the patient and the needs of other individuals who could benefit from organ donation. Approximately 10 years ago the first transplant co-ordinators were appointed and subsequently these co-ordinators have begun to be involved in speaking to the next of kin.

In addition a further trend is developing. Intensive care unit staff are becoming more comfortable with the idea that once brainstem death has been properly established and this has been fully explained to the family then it is not improper for ITU staff to be also involved in the request for organ donation.

A new addition to this process is the establishment of the national organ donor register, which now contains approximately ten and a half million names. The register is steadily increasing at the moment by about a million names per year. Access to this register is available to senior members of the intensive care staff. It is therefore now reasonable to enquire of the register whether the individual patient concerned has registered for donation. If the wishes of the donor are known then the family is much more likely to agree to organ donation. In this circumstance approximately 95% of families will agree to donation if it is clear that the patient was in favour. If the patient's views are not known then between 50 and 70% of families will agree to donation. In this circumstance relatives feel they have to guess the patient's view or use their own judgement and they are often more reluctant.

Approximately one-quarter of potential donors in the UK are now registered on the national register. The mechanisms for registration have widened in scope and include an invitation via driving licence renewal, passport renewal, change of registration with GP or via the Boots loyalty card, which invites consumers to register. Some local authorities also invite registration when sending out information via the electoral roll. This is the so-called 'vote for life' campaign.

If there is no information on what the individual patient's views may have been then the subject of organ donation will need to be broached with the relatives more slowly. It does not appear to matter who does the request, whether nurse, doctor or co-ordinator. The most important factor is that the individual must be comfortable him or herself with the idea both of brainstem death and of organ donation. Gross *et al.* (2000) reported from a community hospital in Switzerland, for example, that not all staff would consent to organ donation themselves (7% refusal) or for a close relative (23% refusal). Members of staff should not be expected to undertake this request if they are not comfortable with both these concepts and if staff are ill at ease they are of course much less likely to succeed in obtaining the family's consent.

UK Transplant (NHS Special Health Authority) is currently studying the views of hospital staff in the UK to transplantation. Drawing on experience in the West Midlands, they have been undertaking a pilot study (2003) on collaborative requesting, i.e. the combination of ITU staff and donor co-ordinator working together. There is some evidence that there is a better response to co-ordinated requests (S. Falvey, Director, Donor Care and Coordination UK Transplant, personal communication, 2003).

One interesting anecdotal observation was reported by an American organ procurement organization (OPO). It was observed that the refusal rate was reduced if staff were employed who had previously been drug representatives, i.e. they had been trained in sales techniques. This background educated the member of staff to be sensitive to the reaction of relatives and therefore to be aware when to push firmly or when to back off for a few minutes and change the subject. This emphasizes essentially the skill and expertise needed in this negotiation. It shows also that one can learn to do it better.

Gortmacher *et al.* (1998) identified three factors likely to increase acceptability of donation requests. Relatives were more likely to agree when the request was 'decoupled' from patient care, in other words when the family understood and accepted brainstem death before discussion on organ donation was begun, when a transplant co-ordinator was involved in the discussion and when the request was made in a quiet and private place.

De Jong *et al.* (1998) also found that families were more likely to agree to organ donation when they had been satisfied with the hospital care that their relative had received and had established good rapport with medical and nursing personnel.

In the past it has been traditional to offer organ donation as an option to the family or as a service without pressure, i.e. a neutral approach. However, nowadays the shortage of organs is so severe, the success rate of donation so good and the public broadly so supportive that a more positive approach is now justified. One should acknowledge that the family may refuse but the presumption should now be that organ donation is a good thing for everyone, for the family, for the recipient and for society in general.

The subject of potential organ donation can be opened by asking the relatives whether the patient carried a donor card. Nurses in the intensive care unit often open the discussion by saying something like 'I wonder if your father/ husband would have wanted his organs donated for the benefit of others'. Nurses also often pick up this issue when it is mentioned in conversation by the family.

Conventionally when attending trauma victims, or now more commonly following brain haemorrhage, doctors wait for brainstem death to be established and especially in the young many healthy organs may become available. Once a patient is brainstem dead even, although they are still being ventilated etc., doctors usually feel comfortable with raising the question of organ donation. The doctor's duty is no longer to the patient since this patient has now died.

At this point it can be helpful to explain to the family that the entire brain has died and that legally the patient is dead. This can be difficult for relatives to accept especially when the patient remains warm and even responds via involuntary spinal reflex and, for example, may move if the hand is touched. It can be useful at this stage to show relatives the results of a CT scan if they wish or to show the EEG report, which describes a complete lack of responsiveness. It can also be helpful to volunteer to involve a neurologist in order to confirm that the patient is genuinely brain dead. Families appreciate a second opinion in these circumstances and it helps them to handle the fact that their relative has died.

When discussing the issue of organ donation the approach usually taken is to suggest that out of the tragedy for this family there can come benefit to others. It can be helpful to ask 'What do you think your mother/sister would have wanted in the circumstances'?

Families can be proud of the generosity of their relative and acknowledge that he or she would have wanted to make this gift.

The importance of this conversation taking place in a quiet, private environment cannot be overemphasized. This is a time for contemplation and an altruistic philosophy. It is also important not to rush these discussions. Some teams call in a transplant co-ordinator early, although others feel that a transplant team should not be involved until the family has clearly begun to contemplate the matter. Often families want to discuss this issue with other family members before reaching a conclusion.

Careful timing and sensitive negotiation is needed if the current shortage of organs for donation is to be addressed.

Withdrawal of active treatment

Many doctors as well as patients find it difficult to accept that there can come a time in the management of patients, especially those who have responded to treatment over a long period of time, when active treatment is no longer either possible or likely to be effective. This does not, however, mean that it is ever appropriate to use the phrase 'nothing more can be done'. Withdrawal of active treatment does not mean withdrawal of all treatment. Rather the emphasis will change from treatment with the aim of cure or prolongation of life to that for relief of symptoms and for the promotion of the patient's comfort and dignity. The phrase 'nothing more can be done' has a desperate ring, which leaves the patient feeling abandoned, anxious, and frightened of dying in pain.

In approaching a conversation about withdrawal of active treatment it is important to stress that it is the aim of treatment that is changing rather than the quality of care. Treatment that up to this point has been designed 'as treatment for living' will essentially transform into 'treatment for dying'.

In explaining this situation to patients and families, it can be helpful to go back over past history and place the severity of the condition in historical context. The patient was faced with this serious diagnosis. The following treatments have been tried and have either failed or were initially successful but are losing their effect. The alternative treatments are either non-existent or inappropriate for good reasons, which are specific to this individual patient. These reasons will probably include the very low likelihood of success, the excessive toxicity involved or the excessive demand on the personal, physical and emotional resources of the patient concerned.

Rarely it will also be necessary to explain that, although treatment may be available at this time under limited experimental conditions or elsewhere in the world, the National Health Service is not currently providing the particular treatment. Resource issues are difficult for patients to accept especially when they are perceived as denying a patient whose life is threatened the opportunity of 'cure' or prolongation of life. Staff of the Patient Advice and Liaison service (PALSs) report that their commonest problems arise from families who feel that their relative is being denied treatment. It is worth knowing also that under the NHS patients and their families do not have the right to demand the institution of inappropriate treatment. The courts have in the past been clear that in the face of conflicting views it is the doctors in consultation with other health-care professionals and managers who have the responsibility for these decisions and that a Local Health Authority and the staff employed by the authority cannot be required to provide treatment against professional advice or at an expenditure that denies others their rightful treatment (e.g. R v Secretary of State for Social Services, ex p Hincks 1979 (Finch 1981), and Re Walker's application 1987).

Ideally the question of conflict will not arise. Having explained the evolution of the patient's condition and the futility of further treatment, it is important to reassure the patient immediately that all appropriate measures will continue to be taken to reduce symptoms, control pain and orchestrate a dignified and comfortable death. At this stage it is important to clarify which members of the health-care team will continue to be responsible for the patient's welfare. Ideally in circumstances where palliative care is appropriate there should be a gradual hand-over of responsibility for the medical and nursing duties to those who are experienced in managing issues that are import-ant at the end of life such as home or hospice care, family farewells and bereavement counselling.

The dying patient

Those who are dying need above all reassurance. They need to know that their symp-toms will be controlled as far as is possible. The emphasis of communication both in word, attitude and behaviour needs to convey the message that the patient is safe and treasured as an individual in their own right. Rarely do patients actually ask 'Am I dying?' but when they do most doctors will try to be truthful but possibly vague. Despite the many and often fiercely held views on life after death none of us who are still alive actually know what, if anything, happens after death. We can only reassure our patients that the circumstances of their dying will be dignified, comfortable and caring.

Opinions vary as to how accurately patients should be told when they are dying. Most doctors believe that the experience of dying is a fundamental part of life and that patients prefer to be alert to this experience and not to be denied the opportunity to say at the end of life those things which pride, jealousy or fear of rejection have pre-vented them imparting earlier in life. Some choose to make confessions, some apolo-gize for past wrongs. Many of us feel that dying is an intensely personal experience, awareness of which no other human being has the right to deny us.

On the other hand there are those who take an altogether different view. They feel that dying is punishment enough and that to inflict the knowledge of his or her imminent death on a frightened, vulnerable patient is an unjustified cruelty. Perhaps there are occasions when parents may seek to protect their children, but in fact most dying patients are aware that they are dying without the need for explicit truth.

A doctor's inability to resolve his or her own personal experiences of death makes empathy much more difficult and is one of the commonest reasons for doctors to appear cold and unsympathetic.

Most of us find death, both our own and other people's, hard to contemplate and each of us seeks to come to terms with it in our own way. It is simpler to define our professional attitude, the essentials of which should be compassion and reassurance.

Advance directives or living wills

An advance statement is a mechanism whereby competent people give instructions about what is to be done if they should subsequently lose the capacity to decide or to communicate. It may cover any matter upon which the individual has decided views but is most often quoted in connection with decisions about medical treatment, especially the treatment that might be provided towards the end of life. It is, in fact, another form of communication and thus included here. The fundamental aim of the advance statement is to provide a means for the patient to continue to exercise autonomy and shape the end of his or her life. This is not a new idea as patients who have been aware of impending health problems have often discussed with their doctors how they wish to be treated. The advanced directive registers these views in a more formal way enabling a patient to influence the provision of treatment as far as it can be foreseen. One obvious problem with an advanced statement is that patients may not have enough information to foresee the circumstances that will arise and may therefore make advanced statements that are contradictory or confusing. For this reason it is strongly recommended that patients who draft advanced statements should do so with the benefit of medical advice. These usually form part of a continuing dialogue between doctor and patient and evolve out of discussions that help to crystallize the patient's personal views.

In practice it is the refusal of specific forms of treatment that usually constitutes the patients most important advance directive. It is a general principle of law and medical practice that all adults have the right to consent to or refuse medical treatment. Advance statements are a means for patients to exercise that right by anticipating a time when they may lose the capacity to make or communicate a decision. It follows that good medical practice will respect the right of people with capacity to be able to define in advance which medical procedures they will and will not consent to at a time when that individual has become incapable of making or communicating the decision. On the other hand the courts have also made it clear that patients can authorize or refuse treatment but cannot make legally enforceable demands about specific treatments they would want to receive (see Re Walker's application 1987). Nor can health-care providers be required to act contrary to the law and so an advanced request for active euthanasia, for example, would be invalid.

The doctor's responsibilities in relation to advance directives

For both ethical and legal reasons doctors must take note of advance statements. It is the patient's responsibility to ensure that where relevant the statement is available to staff involved in their medical care. In practice this usually means lodging a copy of their statement with their GP and drawing this to the attention of hospital staff when appropriate. In hospital you should ensure that a copy is included in the notes and referred to as necessary.

To be incontrovertibly valid an advance directive should contain the following information:

Full name

Address

Name and address of GP

Whether advice was sought from health professionals

Date drafted and reviewed

A clear statement of the patient's wishes, either general or specific

The name, address and telephone number of a nominated (proxy) person if one is given

A signature and witness signature

Although not as definitively binding as written advanced statements, oral expression of firmly held views should none the less be respected. When a patient has intimated clear views on a number of occasions to reliable witnesses, while retaining mental capacity, then weight should be given to these views when considering the decisions that the patient envisaged. Thus competent adults have an established legal right to reject medical advice, assessment or treatment except in cases where this harms others or conflicts with legislation. Doctors who knowingly act in disregard of such competent advance refusals would be likely to be held guilty of assault. Conversely, a doctor who acts in good faith in accordance with an apparently valid advance directive would not be considered negligent. In practical terms it is worth noting that a patient is not felt to be able to refuse 'basic care and hygiene'. It is generally accepted that basic care means procedures essential to keep an individual comfortable. These include provision of warmth, shelter, pain relief, management of distressing symptoms and hygiene such as the management of incontinence.

Doctors on the other hand cannot be obliged to act contrary to their conscience and some have a religious objection to the curtailment of life-prolonging treatment even at the patient's request. Doctors with a conscientious objection to withdrawing treatment should be ready to step aside and ensure that an equivalently trained member of the profession assumes the patient's care.

Breaking bad news

The practice of medicine very often involves breaking bad news to patients. Often the bad news is of a practical and rather trivial nature. For example, this may simply be telling a patient that they need an operation and will have to postpone a planned holiday. There may also be unexpected ramifications of fairly simple bad news. For example, a simple fracture of the ankle may have much greater impact than you expected on a life and career if the patient is an athlete or cause great distress to an amateur runner committed to raising charity funds in a forthcoming fun run! Perhaps surprisingly there is more than a little truth in the observation that the practice of medicine involves communicating 'lots of little bad news every day!'

The term 'breaking bad news', however, usually conveys the necessity to impart the very serious diagnosis of a chronic or life-threatening illness and this topic has been very well covered in the literature. For excellent practical guidance on the conduct of these difficult interviews see Buckman and Kason (1992), Fallowfield (1993) or Faulkner and Maguire (1994). Breaking bad news well requires not only good communication skills but also personal self-awareness, an ability to access the emotional context of the conversation and to be 'emotionally articulate'. The importance of 'pacing' the interview to the needs and abilities of the individual patient cannot be over-emphasized and older patients in particular need time to absorb information.

Before embarking on a distressing conversation, which may, for example, be breaking news of the diagnosis of cancer or a serious degenerative condition, it is sensible to deal with practical issues first. For example, a patient who is attending for the result of bronchoscopy that has diagnosed lung cancer, may well have bone metastases and pain. It is wise to deal with these symptoms first to ensure that these are properly addressed before the patient becomes too shocked and distressed by the impending news to take in the good practical advice given.

In addition to the authors listed above Ptacek and Eberhardt (1996) conducted a review of the literature concerning 'breaking bad news'. Although the recommendations given in the 67 selected references they reviewed were quite diverse they summarized those that occurred repeatedly in these articles. Their recommendations are listed below.

Breaking bad news: what the medical literature recommends

Most medical articles surveyed were clear about the main elements of what patients want from their doctors in these circumstances. Their recommendations were analysed in two broad categories: the physical and social setting and the content of the conversation or 'message' (see box).

Physical and social setting

1. *Location:* quiet, comfortable and private.

2. *Structure:* convenient time, no interruptions, enough time available to ensure no rush.

3. *In person, face-to-face:* make eye contact, sit close to patient, avoid physical barriers.

4. *People:* support, relative and/or nurse, identify and have present at patient's request.

Message

1. *What is said:* preparation, give a warning shot, find out what the patient already knows, convey some measure of hope, acknowledge and explore patient's reaction and allow for emotional expression, allow for questions, summarize the discussion verbally and/or in written form. Consider the role of taping the conversation.

2. *How it is said:* emotional manner: with warmth, care, empathy and respect.

3. *Language:* simple, direct, careful choice of words, avoiding medical jargon or technical diagnostic terminology and avoiding euphemisms.

4. *Give news at person's pace,* allow them to dictate what they are told.

These suggestions epitomize good patient-centred practice and form the essential framework of a common-sense approach to such conversations.

Although the majority of research in this area has focused on the doctor giving information, a few studies have taken into account the receiver's perspective. Of interest is the frequency with which patients volunteered that they would value written information (Ptacek *et al.* 1994).

Patients vary in their response to bad news and it is impossible to predict how anyone will react. Some patients sit quietly and say little or nothing, others become very distressed and others still are angry and agitated. When first faced with the shock of an adverse diagnosis patients will probably be thinking haphazardly and concurrently on multiple levels: 'Why me?' 'Why didn't I go to my GP sooner?' 'Will I need an operation?' 'Will I be able to go on working?' 'Am I going to die?' 'What shall I tell my daughter?'

Most patients prefer to have the support of a friend or relative during these difficult interviews. However, some patients may prefer to face bad news alone and then decide what and how much they will share with their family (Littleford 2002).

Encouraging a patient to bring support with them to this interview carries a number of advantages. First of all the suggestion that the patient may need a relative or friend as support forewarns them that the results of recent investigations, for example, may be adverse. Not only does a companion offer emotional support but they can also often retain more information than the patient themselves as they are slightly distanced from the distressing impact of the news. A companion can also act as a continuing line of communication for the future.

Delivering bad news is of course stressful, not only for the patient but also for the doctor. Medical students in training have in particular voiced concerns not only about how to communicate the news but also about how they themselves will cope with patients' reactions (Sykes 1989).

Doctors may postpone uncomfortable interviews for longer than is reasonable frequently because of the emotional distress that they themselves feel. Alternatively, doctors can feel stressed by being pressed to give information before they are ready to do so. They may, for example, not have had time to research survival information and be in a position to properly advise the patient about the likely prognosis. Doctors feel especially stressed in delivering bad news if they perceive that they themselves carry some blame. For example, if they feel that they have missed or delayed in establishing a diagnosis, they may feel guilt, which increases their sense of stress. However, undue delay provokes anxiety in the waiting patient and in this situation the patient knows that 'No news is not necessarily good news' Better to tell the patient as much as you can and come back when possible with further information.

Delivering bad news in front of colleagues can further increase stress levels. Although it is beneficial for important conversations to take place with the support of other health-care professionals such as nurses with whom the patient is familiar, many doctors feel uncomfortable especially when inexperienced, in breaking bad news in front of colleagues. For the benefit of future patients it is important that junior staff, when appropriate, also attend these interviews, but the requirement for training needs to be balanced against the intimidating effect for the patient of the presence of a number of professional staff.

Doctors who leave a distressing conversation in some discomfort themselves, need to avoid carrying this stress into their next consultation. Take a short break or chat for a few minutes with other staff.

Difficult as it is to break bad news to a patient, it can be equally difficult, for example, to impart news of an impending death to family members. If done badly there may be little or no opportunity to make amends as you may not see the family again and the psychological damage is potentially long lasting.

Following a bad news interview the patient's immediate sense of shock generally gives way later to longer-term stress as the implications of the news sink in. This stress can be characterized as dividing into two forms:

1. What is at stake and what is to gain or lose as a result of this information?

2. What personal resources do I have available to respond and to cope with this stress?

Personal resources can entail family support systems, financial backing and personal skills.

Occasionally the stress of a bad news interview can be enormously increased if there is no 'situational' warning, no 'shot across the bows' either from the doctor or the circumstances. For example, a patient attending for a simple check-up will be ill prepared to face the possibility that an asymptomatic cancer may be diagnosed. In contrast, most patients who attend their family doctor to report a lump will suspect that there is a possibility of malignancy.

An important message, which should not be overlooked, is the value of leaving a patient and family with some degree of hope at the end of these interviews. Even if the outlook is extremely dire there can still be hope in the assurance that comfort and dignity will be maintained and the patient will not be allowed to die in pain. Identifying intermediate, attainable goals such as good symptom control can go some way to mitigate the anxious patient's desperate feeling of powerlessness in the face of overwhelming odds.

However grim the news, you should always be as honest as sympathy will allow. There is no point in wilfully misleading a patient or relative. The truth will inevitably catch up with you and the trust that you have nurtured will evaporate when it is discovered that you have deceived someone.

Careful delivery of news is essential (Stuttaford 2003). Unless the doctor is very careful, patients or their families will allow their imagination to fill in any gaps in their memory created by their shocked inattention. Some may pin their hopes on the one optimistic phrase in a long interview.

Faced with the necessity for a coping effort most patients respond in two phases. First, there will be an attempt to solve the external source of stress and subsequently, with the realization that this is fruitless, an effort to reduce the negative feelings associated with this stress.

Although honesty is to be advocated in most circumstances, Maguire and Faulkner (1988) have argued that euphemisms can be helpful to determine how much information a patient actually wants. For example, faced with the hint of a serious problem most patients prefer to confront the truth and clarify the real position. Some patients, however, cope best by evasion and denial. This is undoubtedly a common and effective coping strategy, which enables many patients to survive emotionally by ignoring unpleasant facts or absorbing them over time at their own pace. If this approach best satisfies the patient's own needs then this should be respected.

One major problem is, however, posed by the adoption of denial as a survival strategy. Many new or experimental forms of treatment for serious illness require explicit consent from the patient and this cannot be obtained without a reasonably realistic appraisal of the patient's situation and the consequent indications for this treatment. It can be very difficult to work out how best to deal with this dilemma. One solution is to put it to the patient as a hypothesis: 'Supposing you were in a very difficult situation and really felt there was no alternative, are you the sort of person who would like to consider some very new or even experimental treatment?' The patient may say 'well yes I suppose if I had to' and you could then lead the discussion on gently to consider the actual alternatives.

On the other hand the patient may say, 'No, I am not going to be a guinea pig and I would never consider it'.

You would probably be wise at this point not to press the patient further but respect their views even if you personally disagree.

The importance of pacing the interview to the needs of the patient cannot be over emphasized. To illustrate the point one example follows:

Patient: This problem that you call heart failure, doctor, it's not serious is it?

Doctor: Well, yes I'm afraid it is. The heart works like a pump and the pump is getting tired.

(Realistic approach)	(Euphemistic approach)
Can I die from this problem, doctor?	Oh, I'm always tired, doctor. You just do the best you can.
Yes, I'm afraid that is very possible. The heart muscle is getting worn out and although we can help a bit with medicine we can't really keep it going much longer.	

In this illustration one patient seeks to grasp the significance of what is happening to him while the other cues the doctor to avoid further details.

As has been noted by others, receiving a serious medical diagnosis may be overwhelming regardless of the care taken by the doctor in communicating the news. On the one hand Persaud (1993) has argued that 'the enormity of the kind of bad news we impart, dwarfs the issue of how it is conveyed to the recipient'. On the other hand the quality of the communication can set the tone for future relations between a patient and doctor and when effective will facilitate the ongoing exchange of information.

These skills may sound intimidating and difficult to learn. Try and identify as you make your way through your early career some 'masters' of communication among senior, experienced colleagues whose style and approach you admire. Spend time with them. Watch and listen. A great deal can be absorbed by 'osmosis'.

Practical tips when communicating bad or sad news

1. If you are called upon to convey adverse news to a patient or family check the patient's notes first. You may have seen many patients since you last saw the person in question and it is essential to have your facts straight.

2. Take the patient or family to a quiet private place.

3. Put aside even a small amount of protected time. It often only takes 10 minutes to break news well. Follow-up visits will be necessary.

4. Leave your bleep at the nurses' station. The nurses understand the importance of breaking news without interruption and will respect good practice.

5. Check that you know exactly who you are talking to, that you are talking to appropriate relatives only.

6. Give some warning of what news is to come. 'I'm afraid the news is not good'.

7. Sometimes in warning of impending death you do actually need to use the words dying and death. You may hope to get the message across without having to be so definite but occasionally you can tell that your message is not being accepted and is not getting through. Although you will not want to cause undue distress, on the other hand relatives may reproach both you and themselves later if they fail to register your message and to support the patient's last hours or days as they would have wanted if they had known.

8. Be very careful about committing yourself to a prognosis. Medicine is full of surprises. Admit to fallibility. Average survival times are known but wide variations are common. Do not be too dogmatic.

9. Take a nurse with you. When you leave it will help the patient if they are not left alone. And if the discussion goes badly you can confer together and try and work out how to do things better.

Breaking news of unexpected death

Usually within the medical context the possibility of death is not wholly unexpected. However, on occasions an accident or acute event may cause death when it was not at all anticipated. Breaking the news of an unanticipated death is a painful and difficult duty. In the case of the patient under the care of a GP or while in hospital, both the patient and their family may be well known to the doctor. More often, however, unexpected death takes place in the Accident and Emergency unit where the doctor may not in fact know either the patient or their family. When, for example, following an ambulance to the accident and emergency unit most families expect their relative to survive in medical hands and rarely fear the worst. Occasionally a family member may receive a phone call out of the blue asking them to come to the A&E Department. Again they may fear serious news but none of us easily embraces the possibility of death.

As with all important conversations it is vital to find a quiet private room where the news can be delivered in a protected environment in a calm and sympathetic manner. The family are likely to absorb from the grave appearance of the health-care team that serious news is impending. It is probably kindest to take the family through the course of events that led up to death giving them time to anticipate the fact that the patient's health problem has seriously and dramatically deteriorated and that in fact death has ensued. Do not delay too long, however, in getting to the point.

When patients are brought in dead to the casualty department or die very quickly in casualty, the main problem in dealing with relatives is their inability to appreciate the rate at which events are unfolding. On occasions the intensive care unit will take in a patient who has no realistic chance of survival in order to give the family time to come to terms with what is happening.

If death occurs rapidly the main difficulty in communication is the problem of answering the family's questions before it is clear what has happened and when no information is yet available. One approach in talking to the relatives is to find out about the patient's past medical history and personal attitude to health. Relatives often volunteer information such as the patient has had heart problems for some time. A family member may say something to the effect that the patient had said that they wanted to 'go quickly'. This gives the doctor the opportunity to say something like 'This may be a shock for you, but in one sense this is what he would have wanted'.

Families may, for example, volunteer that the patient had not enjoyed life recently and that the family can see the death as something of a relief for the patient. It is helpful to let the family volunteer this kind of comment, which the doctor can then reinforce.

Families vary in their response to receiving news of a sudden death. Some want to hear as much detail as possible, others do not. Some simply take the news and just want to leave. The long-term psychological sequelae of this response are probably considerable and relatives should be encouraged if possible to stay awhile and accept support. In a sense the relatives of a person who has suddenly died are themselves acute emotional casualties and as such they become our patients too, every bit as deserving of our care as the person who has died (Marrow 1995).

It is essential that after hearing such devastating news a relative who has come on their own is not left alone and isolated but is offered the comfort and support of a sympathetic team member whose principal role will be that of empathetic listener.

It is also essential after a sudden death to inform the family's GP before 9 a.m. the following day. This forewarns the GP that a death has taken place and enables the doctor to support the family at home. A&E doctors often make the offer to talk again when more information about the cause of death is available after a sudden fatality. In fact, surprisingly, only 5–10% of families take up this option.

Practical tips

1. Leave your bleep at the nurses' station.
2. When called to see the family after a death check the patient's notes. It may be some time after the event that the relatives arrive and you may have dealt with many problems since or may not have been present at the death yourself. Establish exactly what happened.
3. Give a warning of impending adverse news: 'I'm sorry to tell you that things are not good.'

4. If relatives ask who was there when he died never say he was alone. This is often too painful for families to contemplate and engenders futile guilt.

5. It is alright to fall back on clichés. It is comforting to relatives to know that the patient was not in pain, that death was swift, was comfortable, was peaceful.

Multiple bad news

Very occasionally, for example, following a car crash or house fire there are multiple injuries and even deaths within one family. It is possible that a surviving member of the family will have lost not only one or more relatives but also their main source of emotional and cognitive support. For example, tragic accidents can rob a child or adult of the parents or spouse upon whom they normally rely for strength and support in times such as these of injury or distress. Delivering news in such circumstances with multiple serious implications takes great sensitivity on the part of staff. What news to give at what stage, when and how, requires careful timing and support. It can be very difficult to know how much information to give in a single conversation. Sometimes it is necessary to protect the patient from the impact of further complications until the first important fact has been digested. However, excessive delay can lead to the suspicion that the doctor is not being entirely honest with the patient and cannot be trusted.

This dilemma occurs equally when there may be multiple implications arising from a health problem that concerns, for example, a genetic condition or the diagnosis of HIV infection in a newborn baby. Serious neurological conditions, such as muscular dystrophy, can carry profound implications for both the patient and current or future carers. Thinking these problems through carefully ahead of the conversation will help judge the speed at which information can be shared. Nursing and medical staff need to work together as a team and provide the sustained support that will reduce later psychological damage.

Breaking bad news with uncertain prognosis

Most patients and their families prefer to believe that doctors are knowledgeable and well informed and will know enough about the patient's individual condition to advise on options for treatment. It can be very difficult for patients when medical staff are unable to reach a diagnosis or to ascertain exactly what is causing a medical problem. It is confusing and unsettling when there is uncertainty about a diagnosis. It is even more distressing to the patient and their family when a diagnosis is reached without any clear picture emerging as to what can be done to treat the patient and without enough being known about the condition to predict the likely course of events and outcome. Uncertainty is very difficult to accept in these circumstance and patients may be led to seek second opinions far and wide in an attempt to discover whether the medical profession elsewhere in the world is able to provide more information and guidance. These patients and their families are likely to comb the Internet for possible remedies and can be extremely vulnerable to exploitation by unscrupulous advisers or alternative practitioners.

All that you can do as their medical adviser is to be as honest as possible and define to the limits of your knowledge what can be anticipated. Even if no path is clearly advantageous it is probably in the patient's best interest for you to give a lead and make a decision. Suggest the best solution that sensible research has identified. This appears preferable to leaving the patient suspended in doubt and uncertainty. Further clues to the diagnosis may well emerge as time goes by or the effect of your management is seen.

Discussion of medical risks

Many aspects of action or inaction in the medical context carry with them risks. The evaluation and communication of these risks is a fundamental duty of the doctor. This duty arises from the trusting relationship implicit in the doctor–patient interaction and from the duty to promote the ethical principle of self-determination, i.e. patient autonomy.

The concept of risk is complex and difficult to describe. Challenges stem from gaps in the doctor's knowledge about relevant risks, uncertainty about how much information and what kind of information to communicate and difficulties in communicating risk information in a format that is clearly understood by most patients (Bogardus *et al.* 1999). Failure to communicate risks adequately can result in inappropriate decision making, unnecessary morbidity and potential legal complaint.

In order to be useful to the patient information needs to be pertinent both in a personal and medical sense and accessible to the individual person. The concept of risk embodies two distinct notions: first an unwanted outcome, and secondly some uncertainty about the likelihood of that outcome. Bogardus has suggested the terms 'unwanted outcome' and 'probability' to describe these two phenomena.

In discussing a patient's individual situation the questions that you will need to address are as follows:

1. What are the pertinent unwanted outcomes?
2. How permanent is the unwanted outcome?
3. When will the unwanted outcome occur?
4. How likely is the unwanted outcome?
5. Does this result from a single or multiple exposures with cumulative risk?
6. How much does the unwanted outcome matter to this individual patient?

Many of the patient's responses to these questions may be highly individual. For example, the notion that time in the present is more valuable than time in the future is a uniquely personal matter. Such an assessment is fundamental to the calculation as to whether to accept significant present risk for possible future benefit (e.g. side-effects of proposed treatment with a view to increased longevity or quality of life).

In deciding which risks to discuss the doctor must judge whether to address all conceivable risks, the most common risks or only the most important risks. Various standards have been applied to this decision. The 'professional standard' reflects those risks that would be disclosed by a community of your medical peers. The 'reasonable person standard' on the other hand reflects those risks that a reasonable person in the patient's position would want to know. Such a standard appears more in tune with the public's requirement for openness and promotion of patient interests. Generally speaking, serious risks such as death, disfigurement and disability should be revealed as a minimum.

The order in which risks are presented may influence patient choice. The first risk mentioned may not be the most important but may be the only one remembered and may weigh inappropriately in the patient's personal assessment of risk. The tone of voice and choice of language whether factual or emotive can similarly affect the patient's perception of risk.

Qualitative versus quantitative probability

Describing a risk requires a qualitative description but the probability of that risk can be described in two ways. A risk may be verbally expressed as 'rare' or 'common' or alternatively may be expressed as a percentage of likelihood. Some patients prefer qualitative descriptions while others find statistics more helpful. Quantitative data can, however, be value laden in its own way. For example, outcome statistics can be quoted in terms of mortality rates or survival rates. A 10% mortality rate may sound quite different from a 90% survival rate, although the information is essentially the same.

Most people find it easier to understand a risk described as a 'one in ten chance' or a 'one in a thousand chance' rather than more obscure percentages. For example, one in ten of patients having this treatment will need a second course later. It seems to make it easier to evaluate the actual personal level of risk.

Common errors in risk interpretation

Patients often perceive themselves as relatively invulnerable and thus less likely than others to experience an adverse effect (see, for example, Chapter 9—Non-compliant adults). They may give excessive weight to risks they have heard of in the media or be overconfident of the extent and accuracy of their own medical knowledge. In addition it appears that 'new' risks such as SARS (severe acute respiratory syndrome) attract more weight than longer-standing threats. The true perception of risk, as a result, can be skewed.

Reconciling the average and the individual

Perhaps the greatest challenge in discussing risk is to convey effectively an understanding of how the 'average' result may impact on the individual. The average, derived from an analysis of a patient population, may for example suggest a 5% chance of a complication, a relatively low risk. For that individual patient, however, if that complication occurs it is an all or nothing phenomenon, i.e. 100% for them. Reconciling these two concepts requires clarity and explanation.

The process of decision making

Several models exist for handling the impact of risk assessment on decision making. Some doctors behave in a paternalistic way and control the type and amount of information given and ultimately the treatment decisions made. Arguments in favour of this approach stem from the sheer volume and complexity of risks involved and the view that patients inevitably lack the doctor's years of experience and are poorly placed to assess the information for themselves in an informed and balanced way. Arguments against this kind of paternalistic approach stem from the notion of patient autonomy. Alternative models either share the risk evaluation and the decision making between patient and doctor (the ideal) or provide the information and leave the patient alone to decide.

Readily accessible communicators of risk

Many patients find graphic displays more readily understandable than sophisticated numbers (Mazur and Hickman 1993). Alternatively, most people have some idea about common risks in everyday life and some experience of how to evaluate them. Some common risks in the UK were recently quoted in the *Sunday Times* (Leake 2003).
Causes of death in the UK (2001), i.e. risks:

Cancer deaths per year in the UK	190 000
Heart disease deaths per year	132 000
Deaths from influenza	4000
Road traffic accident deaths	3400
Murders per year	1050
Deaths from AIDS and HIV	155

Comparing possible medical risks with these wider risks may be helpful and render medical risks more accessible to normal understanding.

Disclosure of errors

Clinical medicine is a complex business and as with all human endeavour inevitably mistakes will be made. It is essential as soon as a definite error has been discovered that the patient and the patient's family are informed. This task should be undertaken by a senior member of the team. However, circumstances may occur when a junior doctor is the only medical representative present and you may have to deal with the immediate response and call upon your seniors as soon as practicable. It is helpful to understand the overall management of handling the disclosure of errors.

When mistakes have been made patients need to know the exact nature and scale of the error. They need to know the possible implications and long-term effects of such a mistake. They need to know how it came about that the mistake was made and what steps have been put in place to prevent the same error occurring again. Patients want to know that mistakes have been corrected both for their own sake but also for the satisfaction it brings knowing that no one else is likely to suffer the same consequence.

Disclosing that a mistake has taken place and is being investigated and expressing regret that such an event has occurred is not the same as accepting that there has been negligence or that liability has occurred. The question of apologies is covered in Chapter 13.

Accidents do happen and when things go wrong patients understandably feel aggrieved. Mistakes need to be identified and exposed quickly to prevent recurrence but also to defuse the patient's understandable anger and frustration. Patients need to know that lessons have been learned. When something has gone wrong they want to hear that everyone in the team is aware of the problem and what can be learnt from it. They want to know that a full investigation and analysis either has or will be carried out and that steps will be taken or measures put in place that will prevent a repeat. The negative feelings concerning their own problem can be slightly ameliorated by knowing that someone else may have been prevented from being on the receiving end of the same mistake.

Reporting a mistake and apologizing for its occurrence is not tantamount to invalidating a whole medical career. It should not be the doctor's whole professional role that is under scrutiny but only a single mistake or course of events. The doctor's pride, although dented, should not prevent a frank account of what has transpired. Patients usually understand that mistakes are difficult to report and respect the doctor who can manage to explain promptly, sincerely and with a genuine acceptance of the need to learn from the mistake.

When disclosing that an error has taken place it is essential to put aside some time to deal with the patient's natural anxiety and to answer their questions. It is only good manners and is a wise policy to state from the outset that you regret that a mistake has taken place. Many patients say that if doctors had only expressed regret with due humility when first reporting an error then they or their family would have been far less likely to proceed to complaints or legal redress.

References

Buckman, R. (1984). Breaking bad news; Why is it so difficult? *British Medical Journal,* **288**, 1597–9.

Buckman, R., Kason, Y. (1992). *How To Break Bad News. A Practical Protocol for Healthcare Professionals.* Toronto: University of Toronto Press.

De Jong, W., Franz, H.G., Wolfe, S.M., Nathan, H., Payne, D., Reitsma, W., Beasley, C. (1998). Requesting organ donation: an interview study of donor and non-donor families. *American Journal of Critical Care,* **7**, 13–23.

Fallowfield, L.J. (1993). Giving sad and bad news. *Lancet,* **341**, 476–8.

Fallowfield, L., Ford, S., Lewis, S. (1995). No news is not good news: information preferences of patients with cancer. *Psycho-oncology,* **4**, 197–202.

Finch, J. (1981). R v Secretary of State for Social Services, ex p Hincks. In: *Health Services Law,* pp. 37–9.

Gortmaker, S.L., Beasley, C.L., Sheehy, E., Lucas, B.A., Brigham, L.E., Grenvik, A., Patterson, R.H., Garrison, N., McNamara, P., Evanisko, M.J. (1998). Improving the request process to increase family consent for organ donation. *Journal of Transplant Coordination,* **8**(4), 210–17.

Gross, T., Marguccio, I., Martinoli, S. (2000). Attitudes of hospital staff involved in organ donation to the procedure. *Transplant International,* **13**(5), 351–6.

Hope, A. Ethox, The Oxford Centre for Ethics and Communication in Health Care Practice, University of Oxford. Undergraduate course in Medical Ethics: End of Life Issues.

Hope, A., Savelescu, J., Hendrick, J. (2003). *Medical Ethics and Law: The Core Curriculum; End of Life Issues.* Edinburgh: Churchill Livingston.

Littleford, A. (2002). *Breaking Bad News.* Wolverhampton: Compton Hospice Study Centre.

Maguire, P., Faulkner, A. (1988). Communicating with cancer patients: handling bad news and difficult questions. *British Medical Journal,* **297**, 907–9.

Marrow, J. (1995). Telling relatives that a family member has died suddenly. *Postgraduate Medical Journal*, **72**, 413–18.

Persaud, R. (1993). Breaking bad news. *Lancet*, **341**, 832–3.

Ptacek, J.T., Eberhardt, T.L. (1996). The patient–physician relationship: breaking bad news a review of the literature. *Journal of the American Medical Association*, **276**, 6496–502.

Ptacek, J.T., Ptacek, J.J., Dodge, K.L. (1994). Coping with breast cancer from the perspectives of husbands and wives. *Journal of Psychosocial Oncology*, **12**, 47–72.

Times/Law Report (1987). Re Walker's application. *The Times*, 26 November.

Regnard, C. (1994). Breaking bad news: a flow diagram. *Palliative Medicine*, **8**, 145–51.

Stuttaford, T. (2003). Breaking news: we are mere mortals. *The Times*, 1 November.

Sykes, N. (1989). Medical students fears about breaking bad news. *Lancet*, **564** (Letters).

Way, J., Back, A.L., Randall Curtis, J. (2002). Withdrawing life support and resolution of conflict with families. *British Medical Journal*, **325**, 1342–5.

Chapter 7

Dealing with strong emotions and difficult personalities

Peter Maguire and Carolyn Pitceathly

Summary

Doctors tend to use strategies to distance themselves from patients and relatives who manifest strong emotions. This chapter examines the reasons for this distancing behaviour and its effect on patients. Strategies are discussed that can help deal with patients who are angry, distressed or withdrawn. When doctors are faced with patients whom they perceive have difficult personalities there is a danger they will react negatively and dismiss the patient as unreasonable, and uncooperative. Techniques are discussed that can help manage those difficult patients who manifest dependent, histrionic, narcissistic, obsessional-compulsive or borderline personalities.

Dealing with strong emotions

When doctors encounter patients or relatives who express strong emotions such as anger, despair or distress they often feel uncomfortable. They tend to respond by employing strategies that are designed to keep these emotions at a distance. Thus, they may try to normalize the distress experienced by the patient after diagnosis of a serious illness by saying that distress is normal in the circumstances and wholly understandable. This is designed to educate patients that the levels of distress they are experiencing are not something they should be concerned about. This normalization effectively blocks patients from disclosing further emotions and the concerns provoking the distress. When serious concerns about illness and treatment remain undisclosed patients and carers are at high risk of developing clinical anxiety and depression.

Studies of breaking bad news in the context of cancer have found that when patients become distressed on assimilating the news most doctors try immediately to counter this distress by fostering hope. They do so in a genuine belief that hope is essential for the patients' psychological well-being. Thus, the moment patients begin to become distressed doctors seek to reassure them that something can be done to help them and the situation is not as bad as it might seem. Such reassurance is premature because the doctors have not yet elicited what the patients' actual concerns are. The reassurance and information that is given are not then tailored to what the patient is actually concerned about or their needs for information. Instead, they are based on the doctor's assumptions about their concerns. This can result in patients perceiving they were given too much information or too little. This puts them at risk of becoming clinically depressed and anxious.

Patients experiencing serious physical illness who become distressed within consultations usually give both verbal and non-verbal cues about their concerns. They may say 'my breathing is worse' or 'I am devastated that I am getting worse'. Instead of acknowledging and clarifying these emotional cues when they occur doctors tend to selectively attend to cues about physical aspects of the illness or treatment ('tell me more about your breathing'). This allows them to avoid getting into strong emotions.

When they encounter more negative emotions such as anger there is a strong probability that they will become defensive, try to justify their position or even begin to withdraw emotionally from the patient. Yet, such defensiveness increases the risk of formal complaints and subsequent litigation.

Reasons for distancing from strong emotions

Doctors readily admit that they avoid acknowledging and exploring patients' emotions because they are frightened that patients will get too upset. The doctors will then not be able to contain the distress. This could harm patients psychologically, result in consultations becoming overlong, and disorganize clinics. Occasionally, doctors suggest that encouraging patients to talk about their feelings about adverse events like, for example, needing a colostomy, will increase the chances that patients will not cope with their predicament and could become suicidal. In reality, the opposite is the case. Allowing patients to talk about their predicament and concerns, providing they wish to, is perceived by patients and carers as therapeutic and usually eases the emotional burden they experience.

Doctors worry that if they explore and then understand the patient's predicament and associated feelings they may get too involved emotionally and be in danger of overidentifying with what their patients are experiencing. They fear this will be too upsetting personally and could threaten their own emotional survival. They also worry that if they show a real interest in how the patient is coping the patient will ask them difficult questions, for example, 'am I going to get better?', 'am I dying?' or 'why wasn't my illness diagnosed sooner?'

Their worries about personal survival are justified given there are data that show that over 25% of senior cancer doctors, for example, had high burnout scores when assessed with the Maslach Burnout Inventory. These doctors reported that they felt emotionally exhausted, had become detached and depersonalized as a way of trying to cope with their patients' feelings, and felt they were accomplishing little professionally.

Problems posed by difficult 'personalities'

When doctors are faced with patients who they perceive have difficult personalities there is a danger they will react negatively and dismiss them as unreasonable, and uncooperative. Doctors may then judge that they are unlikely to respond to help. There is a serious risk that they will also devalue any symptoms of physical and mental illness. Thus, when psychiatrists diagnose patients as having an 'hysterical personality disorder' but these patients also have symptoms of clinical depression, psychiatrists are unlikely to rate the patients as depressed; this is because they devalue these symptoms in the presence of their diagnosis of personality disorder. While patients with difficult personalities may evoke unhelpful responses and judgements there is also a danger that they will provoke excessively positive responses. Thus, demanding and dependent patients may be able to secure too much of a doctor's time at the expense of other patients. They believe that the same excessive amount of time should be given to them throughout their career as patients.

It is, therefore, crucial that doctors are aware of strategies that can help them deal with patients and carers who express strong emotions and patients who present with difficult personalities. These strategies are now described.

Techniques for dealing with strong emotions

The patient who is very distressed

Patients and carers may become obviously distressed when they are given bad news about their diagnosis and treatment. This can be hard to deal with even though it is expected. It is even more difficult to deal with when distress emerges suddenly and unexpectedly during the course of a consultation; for example, when feelings about a recent bereavement are triggered.

It is tempting to respond by reassuring that their distress is normal and they will soon get over it. However, these strategies do not allow patients to express their distress or disclose the concerns that the doctor cannot anticipate.

For example, in the course of a consultation a 45-year-old man with ischaemic heart disease was talking about his fears that he would die soon because three of his brothers had died from heart attacks before they were aged 50. As he was describing these events he burst into tears. The doctor talking to him assumed that his upset was related to his own fear that he would die similarly from heart disease. However, the reality was that he had been badly affected by the death of one of his brothers and had still not resolved his grief. Questions about his own fears triggered this grief and made him feel desolate. So, the question is how can doctors respond differently to distress?

The first step is to acknowledge the distress openly. So, you could say 'as we are talking about your brothers dying from heart disease I can see you have become very distressed'. Instead of making assumptions about why this is you should ask 'I could assume I know why you are so distressed. However, it would help me if you could tell me exactly why you are so upset at the moment?' This allows the patient to say

> I keep thinking about what happened to my brother, Derek. He was taken ill very suddenly with chest pain. We had to call an ambulance. Just before the ambulance arrived he started coughing up blood. He was terrified that he was dying. When the ambulance men tried to get him into the ambulance he resisted them lifting him into it. He appealed to me for help. It was terrible. Eventually I got into the ambulance with him but he died on the way to hospital. Although I am also frightened that I could die from a heart attack I just can't get over the fact that he died in that way. The feelings I experience are just as strong as they ever were. I feel just as bad as when he died.

This passage of dialogue shows that active eliciting of reasons for the distress has been helpful to the clinician. They have suggested an unresolved grief reaction rather than more distress about his own risk of premature death.

It may seem banal to a patient who has just been given bad news about serious illness or disability for the doctor to acknowledge their distress and invite them to give their reasons. For the patient may consider the reasons should be obvious. However, every patient and carer is an individual. It is important not to make assumptions about what their concerns might be. Instead, you should enquire about why they are so distressed after acknowledging their emotional response. If they become angry and say 'surely you know why I am upset' you can respond by saying 'well obviously I have seen many patients in this situation. However, everybody is an individual and it is important I find out exactly what is upsetting you at this point rather than make assumptions. I should then be in a better position to help you'.

Contrary to doctors' predictions this act of invitation to patients to talk about their distress and the reasons for it usually eases the intensity of their feelings and allows them to begin to get their head around their predicament. Far from increasing the risk they will become psychologically disturbed it makes it more likely they will cope with the problems they are encountering.

Handling anger

When patients or relatives become angry it is tempting to become defensive and explain why their anger is not justified. Such responses only serve to intensify the level of the patients' or relatives' anger. Instead, doctors should try to remain calm and respectful. They should acknowledge that they have noticed they are angry and invite them to explain the reasons for their anger. It is very important to encourage them to explain all the reasons for their anger. If some issues are left unexpressed the anger is less likely to resolve.

As they are allowed the opportunity to ventilate their anger and the reasons for it but the doctor remains calm and respectful it is likely that the level of their anger should lessen in intensity. The patient or relative realizes the doctor is taking them seriously and genuinely want to understand what their anger is about. There should then be a transition point where the dominant emotion shifts from anger to some other emotion such as distress or despair that whatever they do is not going to stop their loved one dying from their disease. Most anger is rational in the sense that it is justified by what patients or relatives have experienced. So, it should defuse when these strategies are used.

Sometimes anger seems out of all proportion to the reasons given by the patient or relative. When doctors acknowledge their anger, invite them to express it and explore the underlying reasons the anger remains at a high level instead of defusing. A strategy that may then help is to point out that despite eliciting and listening seriously to their reasons why they are angry, their anger has not lessened. The doctor can then suggest, constructively, that it could be that their anger is being fuelled by other experiences belonging to the past. While the doctor does not know what these experiences are it could help them to reflect on that as a possibility.

Most patients can identify where this additional anger belongs as in the following example.

> *Doctor:* As we have been talking I have tried to encourage you to say how angry you are and why. You are extremely worried that your daughter may not be getting optimal treatment while she is on the ward. Despite our conversation you seem just as angry now as when we started. I get the feeling there could be something else that is making you angry that maybe you do not realize and it belongs to the past. Could there be anything like that?

> *Mr Bowden:* I have been terrified that my daughter will be neglected while she is in hospital and die. I was beginning to be convinced that the staff here did not care about her and she was at great risk. I have just realized that this is what happened to her sister 5 years ago. She was admitted to Accident and Emergency with a fever. I was told she just had a temperature and was fit to be sent home. I accepted this. However, in the next few days she became very ill. She had a very high temperature, looked pale and became breathless. When I took her back to Casualty they did a blood test and told me she had leukaemia. She died only 3 weeks later. I am terrified similar mistakes are being made this time with the care of my daughter.

It may seem surprising that people can put such bad experiences into a compartment and forget them when something else is happening of a similar nature.

Sometimes, despite doctors' best efforts to explore patients' or relatives' anger and invite them to introspect where it may come from they remain very angry. It is important then to consider that the patient or relative might be pathologically angry because they cannot connect with relevant previous issues or suffer from alcohol or drug abuse or some concomitant mental illness such as depression, mania or schizophrenia. In talking to such patients or carers it is crucial to set limits and let them know what behaviours are not to be tolerated. If doctors feel under personal threat they should get help from security personnel. If they are dealing with such angry patients on a regular basis there should be a panic button available in the consulting room.

The withdrawn patient

Doctors find it hard to deal with withdrawn patients who do not seem to wish to get into dialogue with them. It makes them feel helpless and redundant. Thus, a patient a doctor is trying to interview may look away, hide behind a book or simply lie on his bed with his eyes closed. When the doctor asks him how he is getting on he may just grunt and give monosyllabic answers.

As soon as it becomes clear that he does not wish to get into a dialogue it is important to acknowledge this and say: 'I can see we are having difficulty getting into a conversation, I am here to try and find out how you are getting on but, as I say, we are finding it difficult. Can you bear to tell me why this might be'?

Patients in this situation will usually gives clues as to the underlying reasons even if they do not wish to talk at length. Common reasons include patients feeling hopeless and helpless, feeling very anxious, feeling very depressed, feeling angry, patients who are confused, patients who are paranoid and patients who just feel too physically ill to get into conversation.

Patients' responses to acknowledgements of the difficulty in establishing dialogue will usually indicate which of the categories they come into. It is then important to acknowledge what they are saying and comment, for example: 'You say you feel hopeless and there is no point in talking', 'Can you bear to say why you feel like that'? The patient may say 'talking is not going to stop me dying is it'. You can then respond 'no you are right, talking will not stop you dying but if we talk and identify what you are concerned about it may be that talking will help you feel less awful than you are feeling at the moment'.

Where acknowledgement and exploration have signalled that there are important underlying reasons, such as anxiety, depression, hopelessness, and confusion, it is important to explore whether key signs and symptoms are present so that an appropriate diagnosis is made and a management plan determined.

Dealing with strong emotions can be difficult but managing patients and relatives with difficult personalities can be more taxing.

Difficult personality types

Dependent personality

Patients with this personality type find autonomy extremely difficult. They seek to rely on other people for all their needs and try to select out people who will provide the necessary high levels of emotional support they require, and make key decisions for them. When they are unable to obtain this level of help and support they feel abandoned and become angry and even more demanding.

The underlying dynamic is that they are genuinely terrified of having to cope alone. They have no confidence they can cope without leaning on other people. They actively seek the help of others even to the extent that it makes people reject them because they cannot cope with their demands.

Such patients can be emotionally appealing to doctors when they present by saying things like 'you are the first person who has ever understood me or given me time. If we had more time I think I would get better'. This can lead doctors to give them an undue amount of time compared with other patients. If doctors give in to these demands, for example, offering longer and longer interviews or more frequent appointments, the patient becomes increasingly dependent and have even greater expectations that their needs will be met. The doctors will then begin to feel fed-up with the amount of time they are devoting to these patients, the lack of real progress in terms of symptom reduction and the drain on their emotional reserves. Yet, to suddenly end the relationship can lead to major problems with patients becoming angry and/or litigious or threatening suicide because they cannot cope.

It is far better to recognize the potential dependency of such patients as soon as possible and relate to them accordingly.

It is important to educate such patients that while you are willing to do your best to help them with their problems the amount of time you have available is limited because of other demands on your time. This does not mean you are trying to reject them but you do have a defined amount of time that you can spend with each patient. Attempts to get you to contact them by phone between appointments or arrange extra appointments should be met with a firm refusal unless there are very special circumstances.

When firm limits are set like this potentially dependent patients may feel upset and perceive it as a rejection. For example, a dependent patient might say towards the end of a consultation negotiated to last the usual amount of time (say 30 minutes) that she has an important problem to discuss and she needs more time. It is tempting for you to give her extra time. If you do, you are educating her that you are willing to do this on other occasions. Similarly, if no time limits are set at the outset of the consultation dependent patients may believe they have unlimited time. Having a 2-hour assessment interview on first contact with a health professional leads them to expect this every time.

It is most important, therefore, for the doctor to say 'we did discuss the amount of time available today, namely 30 minutes. Our time is nearly up. I would like to summarize what we have discussed up to now and negotiate when we meet next'. If the patient still insists there is something important to discuss the doctor should indicate that it should be brought up at the beginning of the next interview if it is still a major priority. An exception to this rule is when patients disclose belatedly that they could be at risk of a life-threatening physical illness, suicide or homicide. The degree of risk needs to be assessed and appropriate action taken.

Histrionic patients

These are people who appear very intense. They are emotionally labile in the sense that they move from feeling very happy to being very distressed. They are usually dramatic in the way they present, and are seductive in the way they dress, walk and talk. However, the underlying dynamic is that they are terrified of intimacy. Consequently, they tend to move in and out of relationships very quickly.

When they experience a threat of intimacy developing in the consultation in the sense that they are being expected to explore deep feelings they may take flight because they are frightened of this. The 'flight' may take the form of becoming very distressed and leaving your room.

When they attend medical interviews they may offer positive compliments to the physician that are inappropriate to the transaction that is occurring. Moreover, they make efforts to present themselves only in the best light.

It is crucial not to be taken in by this seduction and politely but firmly refuse any overtures: 'I appreciate that you asked me for my phone number but I must emphasize that our relationship needs to remain a professional one. I do not think I can be of any help to you otherwise.'

Narcissistic patients

Patients with this personality type feel they want special attention and treatment. They are perplexed if their entitlement to special treatment is challenged. They are intolerant of how the system of doctor–patient consultations actually works. They believe that any rules can be waived to accommodate their personal wishes. They become angry if they think they are being treated like everyone else and even threaten to make a formal complaint. The temptation is then for doctors to change the way they relate to them to give them special care or to refuse any accommodation.

Their behaviour is usually based on the fact that they have very low self-esteem. Their confidence depends heavily on the extent to which they perceive they are admired and respected by other people.

When such patients are angry it is important to check what is making them angry and what changes in their management would make them feel happier. If their requests seem sensible it is important to determine exactly what they want. It might be possible to meet these requests without compromising the overall level of care given. Equally, you should let them know when their special needs cannot be met through practical or other reasons:

> Doctor—you insist that you must be able to talk about your worries with the Consultant on a fortnightly basis. The Consultant has to make sure he attends equally to the needs of many patients. It is, therefore, not possible for him to see you as often as you request. However, we can do our best to make sure you see him on a reasonable number of occasions, is that all right?

Obsessional compulsive patients

These patients are very concerned about high standards and morals. They have a strong conscience but find it difficult to cope with feelings. They find it difficult to tolerate life when their routines are threatened. Their high standards can make them intolerable of the behaviour of other people when they too fall below these standards. They also may have issues around cleanliness and orderliness.

When ill they find uncertainty of treatment or prognosis especially difficult. They feel out of control and worry that 'they will fall apart mentally'.

It is important to acknowledge this and legitimize how the patient feels. So, explain you have some sense of how difficult the uncertainty is for them given that they are people who have always organized their lives. When it is possible they should be given markers of progress carefully and accurately. When it is impossible to give them such information this should be acknowledged.

Their information needs should be established by asking them exactly what information they would like at each key point in their illness. They should also be invited to make choices about treatments where such choices are possible. If choices are not possible they should be given careful explanations about why this is not so.

When patients with such personalities remain frustrated it is important to acknowledge this: 'Whatever I try to tell you, you still seem frustrated, could you let me know exactly what you want from us.'

Borderline patients

Some patients present with a history of unstable personal relationships, rapid shifts in their mood and impulsive behaviour. They usually swing between intense affection and love and hatred of their loved ones. The same pattern will usually show itself in relationships with health-care professionals. They suffer from rapid mood swings and go from being cheerful to being very down. They find it heard to be alone, have problems in completing tasks and give in to their impulses even when socially inappropriate. The underlying dynamic is that they feel unloved and are easily threatened by people and circumstances.

Paradoxically, their behaviour often leads them to be rejected, which is what they most fear.

They tend to recreate this tragic circle of neediness, rejection and bitterness in their relationships with doctors. Thus, a doctor may be confronted with a patient who one day admires her and speaks to her in glowing terms. On another she says very negative things about her. It is important to recognize that such patients have little insight into their behaviour. They find it easier to blame other people for triggering their emotional reactions and behaviour.

The key thing to remember is that the borderline patient is very fearful of relationships and expects to be let down. They have deep and continuing needs for reassurance. It is, therefore, important to try to provide support and reassurance at a reasonable and consistent level but also set limits in terms of what can be addressed in terms of the patients' concerns and fears.

Sensitive attention to their underlying fears can enable health professionals to communicate well to support and facilitate a better adaptation in the patient.

It is best to try and provide consistent support through assigning key members of staff to their care rather than allowing inconsistency of care. Teamwork is also important to manage splitting when such patients allege that some medical practitioners are good and others bad.

Conclusions

Use of the suggested strategies will help lower the levels of emotion and difficult behaviours to a point where patients and relatives become more manageable. However, doctors should resist the feeling that they must try to fix the problem unless they have had appropriate training. Instead, they should consider getting advice from or referring on to a senior medical colleague, specialist nurse, counsellor, psychologist or psychiatrist.

Handling these situations can be emotionally draining and leave doctors with feelings of inadequacy, being out of their depth and deskilled. Ways of dealing with these feelings are discussed in Chapter 15 on maintaining a balance.

Chapter 8

Difficult conversations with children and parents

Melinda Edwards

Summary

Although effective communication skills are a pre-requisite in all aspects of clinical medicine, paediatric care can present unique challenges given the need to work with both the family system and health care system in issues regarding the responsibilities and welfare of the child. In addition there are the challenges of communicating complex and sometimes very emotive information to children within a range of cognitive and developmental maturity.

Effective communication therefore requires a systematic perspective, listening sensitively, respecting the views of the family and health-care team and striving to achieve a shared understanding of the best interests of the child. A developmental understanding of children's cognitive and emotional maturity is necessary for deciding how to disclose information. Finally, effective communication is a skilled process which requires time and careful planning.

Introduction

It is not possible to predict or avoid all situations or discussions that may be problematic, emotive or stressful. It is possible, however, to identify good general principles for effective communication that might help at these times. Good communication enhances the quality of the child and family's relationship and satisfaction with the health professional team, as well as having an impact on their subsequent coping and adjustment with the medical challenges being faced. Effective communication is also important from the perspective of the health-care professional, who can hopefully gain some comfort from the knowledge of having handled these difficult conversations as helpfully and sensitively as possible. The chapter will aim to identify the most likely sources of difficulty and consider helpful strategies for managing these conversations with children, young people and families. Throughout this chapter any reference to parents should be assumed to refer to people with parental responsibility for the child.

Difficult conversations within paediatric medicine can arise as a result of challenges in the followings areas:

1. Caring for the child in the context of his or her own family; respecting and supporting the rights, needs and wishes of children while understanding and respecting those of their parents, siblings and wider family system.

2. Communicating important and sometimes quite complex medical information to children and young people across a wide spectrum of cognitive and developmental maturity.

3. Communicating information that is highly sensitive or distressing—there is nothing more emotive than the suffering or possible loss of a child.

Communicating with the child and family system

Children cannot be considered in isolation, they exist as an integral part of a family system. Their behaviour and well-being can have a major impact on family functioning and they can be profoundly affected by other family members in terms of the coping resources and support provided. In the majority of instances, family are the greatest source of support for the child and will have the best knowledge and understanding of his or her needs. It is therefore always important to be respectful and facilitative of the family's supportive role and not to undermine the family system. The aim is to try always to work in partnership with parents, sharing knowledge, experience and expertise relating to the child and the medical situation in order to jointly plan and provide the highest quality of care. Children do not play a passive part in this process. A further aim should be to develop a relationship with the child or young person in which their rights, needs and wishes are understood and respected, and where children are enabled to participate as fully as they would wish in treatment plans, with due respect to their developmental and cognitive maturity (Edwards and Davis 1997).

It is normally assumed that all those caring for children will have the child's best interests at heart and so it can be a time of immense stress and frustration when the family and medical team disagree and have different views on what is in the best interest of the child. Important areas of potential disagreement include the extent to which children are informed and involved in discussions about their treatment, and different opinions about appropriate medical treatment and issues around consent. Each of these areas will be considered in turn.

Involvement in treatment discussions/decisions

Although best health-care practice promotes active involvement of young people in decision making affecting their care, parents may have a number of different reasons for not wanting to inform or involve their children in medical discussions. It is important to try and understand these reasons, working with parents to explore the consequences of excluding or including children in this process and the possible options that are available to them. It is not advisable to just challenge or override the parents, as undermining them at this point will serve to compromise the support they are able to provide for their child, both at the current time and in the future. If parents or carers feel unable to support their child in knowing certain information, then disclosure of this information may not yet be in the child's best interest.

Often, parents want to protect their child from very upsetting news as they consider this an intolerable burden of 'knowing', which they feel might destroy the innocence of their childhood or at worse lead to total despair and the child giving up his or her will to live. Given parental experiences of feeling overwhelmed and devastated at this time, it is perhaps not surprising that many want to protect their child from this. It may also be that parents are feeling so undermined in their parenting role that they feel inadequate and deskilled in how to give this information to their child or even how to provide support and contain the distress that their child might experience at this time. Furthermore, certain cultural and family norms would exclude some children from being given important information or being involved in decision making. It may be considered to be the role and responsibility of the parents or elders of the family to make all decisions and for this not to be questioned by the children.

Whatever the reasons, beliefs or family norms, it is important for the health-care team to try to join and work together with the family, to come to some agreement about what would be helpful for the child or young person to know and how to support the whole family most helpfully in this process. It may be, for example, that providing enough time for family members to talk through their feelings will help them to prepare and compose themselves sufficiently to meet their child's needs. Providing information to parents about available support for themselves and their child can also be reassuring and empower parents to involve their children more. Support might be in terms of helpful strategies for giving information, including being able to respond to children's questions. Parents may also want to consider who should talk to their child and give this information. Some parents may want to tell their child alone, or joined and supported by the doctor or other health professionals. Others may want the doctor to speak to their child but also be present themselves. Support might also be offered in the form of counselling for the family and the child, to be able to reflect on their feelings and to mobilize the resources they require to be able to cope at this time.

It may also be helpful to discuss openly with parents the consequences of withholding information. For example, if children are not given information they need from the medical team or their family, they may seek and acquire information from many different sources (books, TV and the internet, for example) or from other children and adults, either directly, or as a result of overheard conversations.

> One parent, in an effort to protect her child, was clear that her child Tom, could only be told he was having X-ray treatment for a 'lump' and constantly reassured him in these terms. Tom was involved in many conversations with other children on the ward who talked about having the same treatment, radiotherapy, as they had a tumour. He could also read from the hospital signs that he was visiting the radiotherapy department. This

acquired knowledge was particularly frightening, as he felt confused and alone, feeling unable to talk openly with his mother about what was happening, as he realized she had deliberately withheld this information from him.

Gaining information in an unsupported and *ad hoc* manner will enable less opportunity for addressing worries and misperceptions. It can lead to children feeling alone and deeply troubled by what they know, or think they know, as well as what they fear but do not know. Children's imagination and fantasies about what is happening to them can often be more frightening than reality. Providing information in a structured, helpful way with opportunities to clarify information and to gain appropriate support can go a long way in reducing anxiety and helping children feel their situation is more manageable (Rushforth 1999).

The importance of appropriately involving and informing children relates both to their immediate needs, in terms of gaining some sense of control over their situation and also for their long-term health needs and relationships with those caring for them. The quality of the relationship that is formed with the health professionals will have a significant impact on their confidence and co-operation with future treatments. An important base for these relationships is trust, which is dependent upon honesty and respect in all aspects, including information sharing. There is always a concern that children who have had information withheld or have been misinformed, will at some level feel betrayed and mistrustful of those caring for them, even if this information was withheld for what seemed to be good intentions.

Children also have rights, legally, morally and ethically. Children's rights to expression and receiving information have been clearly outlined by the UN Convention on the Rights of the Child (1989) and the Human Rights Act (1998). One of the key messages from the National Service Framework (NSF 2003) is that children should be encouraged to be active partners in decisions about their health care and to exercise choice wherever possible—although the degree of children's involvement will largely be determined by their competence and maturity (BMA 2001; DOH 2001). Children's rights can be described along a developmental progression as follows.

1. The right to information to know what is happening.

2. The right to express a view.

3. The right for this view to influence decisions made by adults (linked to the child's age and ability).

4. A right to participate fully in decision making.

Children's rights and wishes for information are separate issues. Although children have a right to know, they may not want or need to know. Children's wishes for information may vary on a continuum from not wanting to know, or be involved in any way, to wanting as much information, participation and control as possible. Advocating for children's rights while remaining sensitive to their actual needs and wishes is therefore paramount.

It is also helpful to highlight to parents that giving children information is not an all or nothing event, but a process, which can be built upon over time. This may be particularly relevant where the timing of giving information presents a dilemma, such as when children have degenerative conditions in which symptoms or problems may present at a later stage of life. Partial disclosure of information, providing practical information or attending to children's immediate informational needs can still be helpful and can form a step in the process of children acquiring more complex or comprehensive information.

> The parents of a young boy with Duchenne muscular dystrophy explained to him that his condition, muscular dystrophy, meant that his muscles did not work properly. They were clear they would only wish to give further information to their child over time, appropriate to what he specifically asked and wanted to know.

Another example might be young children with HIV being told that they are taking medicines to help the good things in their blood fight off the germs or the bad things. Further information, including the name of the diagnosis might be given at a later stage, when the child has been able to understand issues surrounding the sensitivity of the diagnosis and implications for telling others about this.

The challenge may be in balancing children's immediate needs for information with what parents feel able to discuss, respecting the very real difficulties facing parents at this time. It is important to be as open and honest as possible with young people, within the framework of information which is permissible to share. It is always easier to build on truthful, basic facts than to retract or change misinformation. A more detailed discussion of how to present sensitive or emotive information in partnership with parents is given later in this chapter.

Disagreements about treatment

A similar process of exploring concerns, informing parents and trying to work in partnership with parents applies when there are different views regarding the most appropriate treatment. This situation may be more likely to occur when the outcome of treatment is uncertain, or when parents are insisting on further medical investigation or treatments, when the medical view is to discontinue tests or to withdraw active treatment. It may be, for example that previous medical investigations have not revealed a medical cause for the symptoms and results suggest that a more psychological approach, based on symptom management and rehabilitation (rather than medical treatment) is most appropriate. Families may, however, be very frustrated that medical investigations have not 'found' the cause and can be concerned that a referral for psychological intervention means their child's symptoms are not believed by their doctor or are considered to be just 'in the mind'. They may also fear that the actual cause has been missed and only further or repeated testing could uncover the reality.

In these situations it is extremely important to give sufficient time to enable the parents (and child) to voice their concerns and beliefs about what is happening. As well as explaining the purpose and result from investigations, these concerns and beliefs need to be addressed thoroughly along with the most helpful plan for moving forward. It has also be extremely helpful to promptly involve the multidisciplinary team, including physiotherapy, occupational therapy and paediatric clinical psychology, to begin developing a relationship with the family and engaging them in a management plan. Good communication between health professionals and the family's GP can be valuable in rationalizing the family's access to medical services and to prevent 'shopping around' for more investigations, and also to utilize the very key role and relationship the GP may already have with the family to help them better understand the medical view.

Second opinions may need to be sought when resolution cannot be achieved and families are demanding continued active treatment when this is not considered to be the most appropriate plan by health-care professionals. As a final resort the courts can be asked to decide what is in the child's best interest. Relationships between the family and health-care team can become very stressed as a result of this level of disagreement, and it is very important that the emotional needs of the child or the family are not neglected at this time. It is good practice to be as open and informative as possible with the family, so they have a comprehensive understanding of the medical and legal process involved. Whenever possible, a member of the health-care team should be identified who can be a support and advocate for the family. It may also be highly appropriate for the child to have a separate advocate and support. Even where there is conflict surrounding the most appropriate medical plan, it will hopefully still be possible to 'join' with the family in agreeing the most helpful way of supporting their child psychologically at this time.

In situations where there is disagreement between parents or other family members, the medical team need to be clear about what they feel is in the child's best interest and advocate for the child. Consent for treatment is only required from one person with parental responsibility even if another person with parental responsibility does not agree. Resources for families to access psychological counselling can be valuable at this time.

There may also be situations in which there is a conflict of wishes between parents and children or where children are requiring some privacy from their family. Young people are entitled to privacy and medical confidentiality if they wish. It may be necessary both to facilitate and provide opportunities for young people to be able to talk to doctors and others healthcare professionals on their own. Parents may not recognize the need for their child to have this privacy, and even if they did, parents and children may find it difficult to request this or challenge an existing appointment system. Providing such opportunities becomes part of the process of empowering young people to assume increasing responsibility for their treatment and medical care. It is also a way of enabling sensitive issues (such as sexual concerns) to be raised, when young people may not feel able to with parents in the room. Generally, confidentiality should only be overridden when there are clear grounds, such as the risk of significant harm, although the aim would always be to support young people in sharing appropriate information with their family.

In a similar manner, one would ideally be gaining consent from both the child and person with parental responsibility. In situations where children and parents do not agree about treatment, legally the decision of a competent child to accept treatment cannot be over-ridden by a person with parental responsibility. However, if the child refuses treatment, those with parental responsibility may consent on the child's behalf for treatment to be given. There are significant implications of parents and the medical team enforcing treatment on a child who has clearly expressed a wish to not have treatment and every effort to understand and work with the feelings and concerns of the child needs to be undertaken. Where a consensus cannot be reached, and where treatment is potentially life-saving for the child, it may be appropriate to take the ultimate decision-making responsibility to court, so that the parents and medical team are seen by the child as carrying out the legal decision, rather than just imposing their own decision about treatment.

Communicating complex information to children

Medical information can be complex and difficult to communicate at many levels, both because of the complexity of the information itself, and due to the breadth of ages, cognitive and developmental maturity of the children involved. The challenge becomes one of identifying the appropriate level of information for each individual child and being able to clarify and make the information accessible. Medical terminology itself is very much a 'foreign' language and often difficult to translate into 'everyday' language for those without medical training. Some words in a medical context take on a different meaning from their daily use. For example, few non-medical adults would consider any tumour or epilepsy 'benign', or that someone following critical surgery was really 'comfortable'. Families often have their own unique words and language for illness and body parts. Epilepsy may be referred to as 'fits', 'turns', 'episodes', 'wobbles', jerks, 'blank spells', 'dizzy spells', 'shakes' and 'stares'. It is very helpful to use the child and family's own terminology (wherever appropriate) in order to be talking the same language, as unfamiliar words can be either not meaningful or more frightening:

> One young boy was anxious when told by the nurse that he needed some strong medicine because he was 'poorly' but was greatly relieved to hear from his mother that he just needed the medicine as he was 'sick' and would be helped to feel better!

Children will make sense of unfamiliar words they hear depending on their experiences and understanding:

> One 8-year-old girl was devastated to hear from the doctor she had diabetes. This word was totally unfamiliar to her and in splitting the word down into its components, her understanding was that she would die from this 'betes'.

Further complexity arises given that many medical processes are unavoidably described in virtual or metaphorical terms, as they are not tangible or visible. Medical prognoses are often based on predictions and probabilities rather than absolute certainties, and for particular treatments, a range of possible outcomes or risks will need to be outlined. In addition, many of the possible outcomes might be realized months or even years in the future with treatment being prophylactic and not leading to any observable difference, rather than actively improving function or symptoms.

Assumptions are often made that children of a given age will have acquired a certain level of knowledge and will therefore be able to understand particular information. In reality, there can be a wide variation of children's understanding within any age group, which is a result of variance in their cognitive and reasoning skills, their direct or indirect experience of the subject area, and how they have been informed and supported in their knowledge. In addition, misperceptions and inaccuracies if left unchecked can easily be perpetuated and lead to a rather idiosyncratic understanding at any age.

> The parents of one child requiring multiple different tablets each day understood the importance of taking all the tablets but not how they needed to be taken. Following vastly discrepant blood results, the parents revealed they had crushed the weeks' medication together and administered a tablespoon each day.

Just as children develop in their ability to process and conceptualize information, different characteristics in their thinking and abilities to understand their illness and treatment become apparent. This will clearly have important implications for communication with children about medical issues.

Young children have less experience of the world and a limited number of constructs from which to make sense of new situations. Most of their knowledge is acquired through direct experience, and is very concrete and bound to the here and now. Medical explanations of treatment focusing on internal bodily processes will not be meaningful until the child has acquired a concept of 'inside' his or her body. Until such a time, it is more helpful to focus information on what the child can see, hear or feel.

Young children's thinking may seem very illogical and can be dominated by magical or superstitious thought. Children may fear they have 'wished' someone to be ill and this has actually happened, or may believe their own illness has been a result of being punished for some wrong doing. It is important to be very positive with children about their efforts or skills in managing medical procedures and to reassure them wherever necessary that the treatment is to help them and that they are not in trouble or being punished. Children's magical thinking may give rise to an expectation for medicine or surgery to make them better straight away (like magic), and they can be devastated to still be feeling unwell if this does not happen, becoming frustrated and losing confidence in doctors and their parents at these times.

> One young boy believed from what his father had told him that he would be better after surgery (like magic!) and go home. He was so cross, he refused to talk to his father for a whole week while he remained in hospital recovering from surgery.

As children's thinking progresses, logical thought processes become more apparent. Initially these tend to be rather concrete and literal, with children demonstrating limited ability to generalize from one situation to another or to appreciate multiple aspects of one situation. At this level, children may struggle to understand the full implications of the available treatment options and outcomes, particularly outcomes that do not change how the child feels or improves symptoms in an overt way. Children who are concrete and very literal in their thinking, may construe parts of their body (such as heart, kidney, lungs) that are not working properly to be 'broken'. These children may also be baffled as to why they are receiving medicine through a line in their arm when it is their leg that is poorly or 'broken'! Children demonstrating basic problem-solving strategies may have limited and inflexible 'rules' governing their understanding of illness, such as believing all illnesses are caused through contagion, applying this to anything from colds to cancer and broken bones.

With increasing cognitive maturity, young people are able to reason more logically and to think in more abstract terms. They can also begin to explore problems more systematically. Abstract reasoning skills and systematic problem solving is associated with later adolescence.

Clearly, any explanations given to children about their condition or treatment will need to be tailored both to their current knowledge and reasoning skills as well as helping them assimilate new information, which will be helpful for them in terms of understanding what is happening to them. One of the challenges is therefore how to assess the level of a child's understanding to be able to gauge the most effective information to give. It can be helpful to listen carefully to children, to their vocabulary, the complexity of their language and how they comprehend and describe their situation. It is also extremely important to facilitate and encourage children to ask questions as this can be a valuable way of checking and monitoring the sense they have made of the information given. Simply asking children if they have understood is insufficient. Many children will nod to say 'yes' for many reasons other than actually understanding. This may be to please adults, to pretend they understand so they do not appear stupid, or simply to bring to a close more quickly a situation that is stressful for them. It can finally be helpful to ask children to reflect back what they have been told or what it means to them. Asking children how they might tell another child (such as a good friend) about the information can be a useful check of understanding.

It is important to be aware of the child's cognitive capacities both in terms of the complexity and amount of new information as well as the pacing of giving this information. Younger children and those with more limited cognitive skills may require a greater amount of time to assimilate and process the information to be able to make sense of it. It is helpful therefore if information can be well structured and in a coherent sequence that can be easily followed. Information needs to be given in manageable amounts, and repeated or built upon over successive conversations. The pace should be directed by the child with sensitivity to how he or she is responding to this information.

Information needs to be presented in a simple and accessible way; this may be verbally, or visually through pictures, demonstration or play. For verbal information, it is helpful to use words or terms that are familiar to the child and to use the child's own words where possible. Complex words and medical jargon can easily confuse or detract from what is being communicated. There are a variety of helpful children's books that present information about the medical condition, treatment or emotional responses to associated feelings (see Edwards and Davis 1997, for a review). Children with more limited verbal skills, may find information presented visually more accessible. Pictures, videos and adapted toys or models can be very helpful. These are often resources available from the hospital play specialist, who can also be extremely helpful in communicating information and preparing children for medical procedures. There are also an increasing number of helpful web pages that older children could be directed to (see list in References), as well as supported opportunities to meet other young people willing to share information and experiences about the condition or treatment.

It can be very helpful to involve children and parents in the process of compiling information and preparation booklets, as in the following example of a mother helping to produce a photograph booklet for her child.

One 4-year-old child underwent amputation of both of his legs below the knee following a serious episode of meningitis. His mother was very concerned and anxious as to how to tell him what had happened to his legs. A book was prepared with his mother using photographs of a special teddy with bandages on his legs carrying out many of the activities (including physiotherapy, attending school and playing) that this young boy had also been engaged in over the past few days. The storyline in the book was of a teddy who had also been very unwell and had woken up to find bandages on his legs. The book emphasized everything teddy was still able to do as well as acknowledging some of the things teddy was now finding too difficult to do such as walking, as he now needed a wheelchair to get around. In the story the teddy was told by his mother that his legs had become very poorly and could not be made better even though the doctors and nurses tried as hard as they could and used the strongest medicine. As teddy's legs could not walk or run, everyone decided that it would be a good idea to have new legs, special legs that would help him run and play again.

In conversation with the child's mother she wished to be the person to read the book to her child. She had already taken a key role in helping to produce the book, choosing pictures and words that she felt were most appropriate for her child. First, she introduced the little teddy (used in the book) as a special friend and then she chose the time that felt right to look at the book and the story together with her child. Her initial dread at telling her child was turned around to a sense of being in control and in a key position to both inform and support her child at this time.

Children may become distressed or anxious at some of the information they will hear. It is important to be sensitive to this and to acknowledge how the information might be making them feel, before progressing on to giving further information. When children are showing total disinterest in what is happening or what they have been told it implies that natural curiosity has been overwhelmed by anxiety. It is important therefore to be able to address the underlying anxiety rather than to continue offering information or reassurance about this information. If children are anxious or preoccupied they are likely to take in even less information. Therefore, plenty of time needs to be made available, possibly over more than one session, to be able to give children the information they require, and to enable them to assimilate and process this information. Children's distress may not be evident by the child being upset or talking about feelings, it may be shown later in their behaviour. Thinking with parents about how their child may react can help both to normalize the child's feelings and prepare parents to support their child at this time.

Children with learning and sensory impairments

Children with a range of learning, sensory or communication difficulties can be helped to participate actively in giving their views and making decisions about their care, depending on how creative and skilled we can be in giving information in an accessible way. A careful assessment of the child's communication skills is required, as well as becoming familiar with the communication system and tools used by the child. Referral to a speech and language therapist may be beneficial if further help is required. Useful resources are provided by many organizations to aid effective communication (please see Marchant *et al.* 1999 and Morris 2002).

Giving emotive and sensitive information

In this final section, an overview of the process of giving emotive or sensitive information will be considered, with particular attention to the preparation and process involved. Giving distressing information is not a single event, confined to when an initial diagnosis is given, but can occur at anytime such as when the medical treatment or condition changes or further intrudes on the life of the child and family. Although we can usually predict what would be viewed as bad news, it is not possible to do this with complete certainty, and it is therefore important not to make assumptions about the meaning and consequent response to the information given.

It is often most appropriate that parents are given very emotive information first, without their child being present. This can enable time to assimilate the information and to plan how to best support their child in receiving the news. The plan may include who should tell their child, the most helpful way of presenting the information, and what support might be helpful following this. Giving parents this opportunity to think and plan together with the doctors or health-care team can empower them and enable them to regain some sense of control and purpose at a time when they may be feeling helpless, and overwhelmed.

> Following medical investigations, the parents of an adolescent girl requested a separate appointment with the doctor and were informed about her potentially life-limiting condition. They were devastated and extremely fearful of bringing their daughter to the next appointment to be given the news. In talking this through with the doctor, it became clear they felt she would be best supported being told by her mother at home, and then coming back to clinic for an appointment together as a family to ask further questions. Both parents clearly felt empowered at being able to carry this through for their child, feeling able to have some control over the timing and process of involving their daughter.

It can be helpful to consider the needs of children while their parents are talking to the doctors. Children are often very sensitive to cues from parents and medical staff that something important is happening around them and can be very anxious and distressed if their parents suddenly leave them to talk to the doctors. It can be even more distressing if parents return to the child looking visibly shaken but with falsely optimistic smiles and reassurances that everything is going to be fine. It is more helpful to be explicit to children about the fact that the doctors will be talking to their parents and being clear with children regarding who will give them information and when.

Particularly for adolescents and older children it is good practice to clarify with them how they would prefer to hear about their test results or diagnoses and to respect their wishes about this. Some may choose to have family present, others may wish to have a private talk with the doctor or choose for a particular member of the health-care team to be present. Although rights to confidentiality need to be respected, in most cases the parents will be told simultaneously or straight after this conversation with the adolescent.

If information is to be disclosed to the parents and young person together, it is important to address information at the pace and level appropriate for the young person and for them to be as engaged as possible in the discussion. It is important that the discussion is guided by the young person's responses and questions. Assurances can be given to the parents that time will be given for any further questions that they may have at the end of the discussion, either with or without their child being present.

As part of the preparation for discussing information, it is valuable for the parents and health-care team to consider the support required both at the time of disclosing the information and to facilitate the child's coping and adaptation following this event. One person needs to be designated to lead in giving information. It can be very confusing if too many people are involved, as they often use different words or inconsistent phrases to explain what is going to be happening. It is important to try and establish what the child already knows and if possible, what they are expecting to hear. A further aim is to understand the possible significance and impact of the information in context, in terms of the meaning it might have for the young person and their life (i.e. if the child is just about to sit exams, change schools, perform in a school play, go on holiday and so on). Information should be well prepared and structured taking into account any comments from parents that might help frame or explain information in the most helpful way.

When meeting with a child it is very important, however basic, to get the child's name right or if the child prefers to be called by a pet or nickname to use this name. In some families, children's full or proper names are only used when the child is in trouble and this is certainly not the message one would want to be giving at this time. It is also helpful to be explicit about what you are about to do and to give an outline regarding the structure of the conversation. As with giving information in any situation it is helpful to start with what the young person already knows before giving any further information. Before the session is ended it is helpful to have a clear plan with the child about what the next step will be and to frame this in the most positive way possible. It can feel uncomfortable if children become quiet and have no questions or comments. This can be due to the shock on hearing the news, feeling overwhelmed by the information and needing time to consider what this means for them. When children do ask questions sometimes people are perplexed at the focus they might place on something that others consider more trivial. It is very important to be respectful of exactly what the child finds the most pressing or preoccupying for them as this again gives an indication of the impact and meaning the situation has for them in their lives at this time. It may also indicate what the child has grasped and understood from the conversation. Physical comfort and reassurance may or may not be asked for by the child at this time and it may be helpful to suggest to parents that they might move closer to their child or to comfort them if this is not done spontaneously. It may be that parents are feeling so overwhelmed and upset at this time that they are unable to initiate a comforting behaviour that they would otherwise have done.

It can also be very helpful to give some written (or visual) information for the child to take with them even if it is just key words or phrases that might be helpful in enabling the child to retain the information for later and to facilitate discussion with family and friends when at home.

> One adolescent understood that his diagnosis was of multiple sclerosis (MS) and was aware of how he was currently affected by this, but found it difficult to be able to tell others. He found himself on more than one occasion telling people that he had MS, only to be told by

them that he could not possibly have MS as this was something only older people had and that he clearly had ME instead! The young man lost his confidence in telling people what his condition was and began doubting that he had properly understood his doctor.

What might have been helpful was to have some written information about MS that was personalized and described how it affected him. One way of doing this is to think of the questions that the young person or others might have about MS and to role play conversations where he could give answers to those questions noting down helpful words or phrases.

Feedback from appointments where significant information is shared, including the responses of the young person and the plan made with them, should be explicitly communicated to the rest of the health-care team, so that everyone is clear and as consistent as possible in their conversations with the young person and family. Similarly, any updates as new information is gained, need to be well communicated.

Effective communication is a skilled process which requires careful planning and takes time. The benefits of this investment are clearly evident both in terms of the quality of care for families and the satisfaction for the health-care team.

References

British Medical Association (2001). *Consent, Rights and Choices in Health Care for Children and Young People.* London: BMJ Books.

Department of Health (2001). *Reference Guide to Consent for Examination or Treatment.* (www.doh.gov.uk/consent).

Edwards, M., Davis, H. (1997). *Counselling Children with Chronic Medical Conditions.* London: British Psychological Society.

Human Rights Act (1998). London: HMSO.

Marchant, R., Jones, M., Julyan, A., Giles, A. (1999). *Listening on all Channels 'Consulting with Disabled Children and Young People'.* Brighton: Triangle.

Morris, J. (2002). *A Lot to Say! A Guide for Social Workers, Personal Advisors and others Working with Disabled Children and Young People with Communication Impairments.* London: Scope.

Royal College of Paediatricians and Child Health (1997). *Withholding or Withdrawing Life Saving Treatment in Children: a Framework for Practice.* London: Royal College of Paediatricians and Child Health.

Rushforth, H. (1999). Practitioner Review: Communicating with Hospitalised Children: Review and Application of Research Pertaining to Children's Understanding of Health and Illness. *Journal of Child Psychology and Psychiatry,* **40**, 683–91.

UN Convention on the Rights of the child (1989). Genera: United Nations

Web pages for young people to access

http://www.teenagehealthfreak.org/homepage/index.asp
http://www.epilepsy.org.uk/kids/
http://www.cafamily.org.uk
http://www.childrenfirst.nhs.uk/index.php

Chapter 9

Special adult groups

Elisabeth Macdonald

Summary

The special groups requiring a particular approach and appropriate conversation style include adolescents, non-compliant adults, the elderly, the elderly frail, the hard of hearing and the bereaved. Different approaches are needed for each group.

Talking to adolescents

When seeking to communicate with teenage patients it is essential to deal with them as equals. They need to be addressed with respect and without patronizing them. Young people are due the respect and privacy accorded to any other patient and matters of medical importance should be discussed principally with the adolescent together with the parents if the youngster is willing. Younger teenagers, aged 13 or 14, are more likely to want close parental involvement than many older teenagers and these two stages of adolescence may need to be handled differently. Young people have their own hopes and fears and these need to be addressed in a sensitive and sympathetic manner. It is worth remembering that teenagers with serious problems have so far in life had everything going for them and a serious health setback can appear, and in reality actually be, devastating to their entire future.

The setting of conversations with adolescents is important. They need both time and space. However, circumstances can be unpredictable and you may find yourself talking to young people when the setting is less than ideal, e.g. in an open ward or in a busy clinic. In such circumstances if privacy cannot be engineered it is better to make another more appropriate arrangement. Serious conversations should never take place over the telephone. The aim is to be open and supportive but not 'bullish'. The ideal is to be frank, and to give information face to face in the presence of a supportive network of family, friends and nursing staff.

One of the most important factors of all is to give the young person time (Segal Barbara, Consultant Child and Adolescent Psychotherapist, Teenage Cancer Trust Unit, Middlesex Hospital London. Personal Communication 2003). This may mean time in terms of days to come to terms with a diagnosis or prepare for a treatment as well as time in conversation to explain what is happening.

It is not unusual for young people to need the same information repeated on several occasions before they can really take it in. Be patient. Know that young people can't grasp it all at once partly because of anxiety and perhaps also because they may use blocking defence mechanisms. Many of us block out unpleasant facts and this is a common coping mechanism. Take an opportunity to go back and ask them 'Did you understand what I was telling you?' or 'What have you made of what I have said to you so far?'

Young people are often quite perspicacious about whom they will trust and whose information they regard as questionable. They may say for example, 'I don't really like Dr X because I don't really trust what he or she is telling me'.

Young people recognize and trust doctors who are honest with them. They know that these doctors have their welfare very close to their hearts and can be counted on to be frank. Occasionally they may say something revealing to other staff such as 'I am going to see Dr J today and I am a bit nervous because I know that he will always tell me the truth'.

Be as open as you can with your patients and know your customers. Most will want to hear information in the presence of their parents and with parental support. Some older teenagers on the other hand will prefer to be dealt with as an individual and separately from their parents.

As you approach a young person it is worth asking them what they would prefer. Occasionally young people say, 'Oh, I have got enough to deal with about this illness and I don't want to know all the fine details so please talk to my parents'. You can then proceed to do this and make the practical arrangements with the parents' help. Observe the youngster's relationship with his or her parents and consult the parents also. In practice parents play a large part in patient management and this is an immensely traumatic experience for them too.

Avoid the use of medical jargon. It will make a youngster feel excluded from the medical 'club' and build up resentment and even fear (Segal Barbara, Consultant Child and Adolescent Psychotherapist, Teenage Cancer Trust Unit, Middlesex Hospital London. Personal Communication 2003). However, it is quite important to introduce young people to correct medical terminology. They will need to know the name of their diagnosis and the appropriate terminology to describe investigations and treatment. They will hear nurses and radiographers using these terms and this can be frightening if they do not understand them.

Be aware that the adolescent finds themselves in a very strange medical environment and suddenly out of their own context and out of their own world. Establish some recognition of the fact that you realize that they are in an alien environment: 'You must find this all a bit weird and a bit of a change from what you're used to.'

This separation from friends and social life may last a very long time in the case of serious illness. Friends often avoid ill teenagers, not knowing what to say to them, and this is especially true if youngsters looks different or have lost their hair.

Most young people find it very difficult indeed to be treated as a child again. After having an independent life before diagnosis and beginning to establish their own identity they find themselves in an alien environment with their parents hovering over them again. They feel suspended in a strange place without their newly established peer identity. Adolescents can't bear to be treated as children but on the other hand they know they need the support which their parents can give. They feel regressed and infantilized but on the other hand they are aware they need their mother's support. As young people like to say their 'space' is invaded. Adolescents guard their privacy jealousy. Be aware of this frame of mind and sensitive to it. For example, young people feel embarrassed at getting undressed in public. Many would much prefer that their parents too were not present. Check this out with them sensitively to find out what is tolerable for them. Acknowledge that they may not feel comfortable and ask 'Is it alright if . . . . . .'.

Young people, especially boys, often behave with swagger and bravado. This often conceals a very nervous young man. When undertaking painful procedures it is important to acknowledge that, although the young person appears tough and brave underneath, they are terrified. Explain that it will be over quickly but that it is necessary and that you understand their level of fear. Recognize their fear without making them feel foolish and childish. Young people are grateful if their fear is acknowledged.

It can be very helpful to involve a clinical psychologist or adolescent psychotherapist on the ward. Young people may not immediately volunteer much information themselves but often respond when introduced to a psychologist 'Oh I am okay but my mum needs to talk'. It can be very helpful for a psychologist to talk to worried parents as this takes the burden away from the young patient. Often young patients know that they just have to get on with it all themselves but they know that their Mum is not really coping. She may be very anxious, is really not herself and is talking about them to friends. Young people find this very uncomfortable. Learn to observe the relationship with the mother and of course understand that parents are anxious and need your time themselves. Some mothers are very sensitive to the needs of young people but, for example, other mothers are not sensitive to the fact that their son would prefer not to undress in their presence.

Be aware that adolescents have their own life-style and timetable. They often stay up much later than adults and as a result sleep in later. This is normal adolescent behaviour and it is important not to expect them to participate in discussions and activities too early in the morning. If you respect their needs they will respect your instructions. Remember that adolescents are patients but they are adolescents first and adolescence for all of us is a very difficult stage of life at the best of times. Show an interest in what interests them in terms of sport, football, fashion, music, etc. Take a holistic interest in them. Adolescents have needs that are different from adults and certainly different from children.

Teenagers tend to form very effective support networks with each other and managing teenagers in specialized units facilitates mutual support and can be empowering to young people (Teenage Cancer Trust 2003). Sadly, such units are few and far between but there is a growing awareness that adolescent medicine warrants a specialty in its own right, and is very different from either paediatric or most adult medicine.

Adolescents themselves are very unsure as individuals and definitely need boundaries. They need to be made aware of what is appropriate behaviour in a clinical setting especially towards nurses and young doctors. The boundaries need to be both physical and emotional. Do not talk about your own private life. Be friendly but do not give too much away. Talking about your own flourishing personal life can provoke envy and if you confide difficulties this can add another worry to the youngster's own concerns. If you are not careful you may occasionally be drawn in to acting in a way that is not appropriate to your professional role and this makes the professional vulnerable.

This kind of medical practice involves being open, honest, friendly and professional but not overpersonal. Young doctors and nurses tend to get emotionally involved with young patients and this is inevitable. It is, as a result, even more important that boundaries are set and kindly but firmly maintained.

Practical tips

1. Be frank and honest.
2. Be patient and be prepared to give young people time.
3. Be informal but not too personal.

Non-compliant adults

Between the ages of 30 and 60 most adults feel that they are 'in the prime of their life'. Often both their working life and family commitments are busy and fulfilling. With this self-confidence comes an expectation of invulnerability. Many people subconsciously presume that accidents, hardship or illness happen to other people but not to them. This attitude can create difficulties for doctors when consulted by patients who are clearly abusing their own health yet are reluctant to acknowledge this. Some patients who, for example, seek advice about symptoms such as recurring headaches may describe a life-style that is fraught with danger. Such patients are often heavy smokers, overweight and with a poor diet, highly stressed at work and with an unsatisfactory family relationship at home. Convincing such patients that the possibility of stroke or heart attack is a real and genuine danger is a formidable challenge for the health-care professional. One common analogy is to draw the comparison between car maintenance and the human body. Patients can readily understand that to maximize the car's efficiency, it is essential to use the right fuel and to service the machine regularly. In a similar way the body benefits from a healthy diet and regular rest and exercise.

However, the right tone is quite difficult to establish. Excessive censure will drive the patient away and probably intensify the very behaviour one seeks to change. On the other hand gentle criticism combined with realistic encouragement may help create a partnership with the patient in an effort to modify the riskier aspects of his or her behaviour.

People find it hard to accept advice at the best of times. It is especially difficult to hear uncomfortable suggestions not only about life-style change but also in other clinical situations about treatment, which has an impact on working or family life.

Normally healthy adults will not anticipate adverse news and when health problems arise they are often busy, preoccupied and highly independent. As a result they may be unwilling to take advice or spend time on discussion or on necessary treatment. Health appears to them to be a matter of secondary importance. In these circumstances it can be difficult to persuade the patient of the value of an agreed management plan.

It is not uncommon for otherwise well-educated patients to have ill-informed or even idiosyncratic views on health care. Individuals who are in control of the rest of their lives, and often in working positions of considerable authority, may have difficulty ceding the initiative in important matters of health to health-care professionals no matter how well intentioned. Be firm but non-judgemental. Involve the practice nurse and if allowed the spouse and children. Empower the patient and their family and train them to care for themselves. A supportive co-ordinated approach laced with humour and a light touch is your best bet.

A further difficulty in dealing with individuals used to authority stems from the patient's perception that it is necessary to be robust if not downright aggressive in order to get the best service from the doctor. The patient may have been kept waiting before the consultation or have encountered other apparent slights. They may start off in a demanding or truculent tone. This usually dissipates if you adopt your normal business-like professional approach. The aggression usually disappears when you demonstrate genuine appropriate concern for the patient's symptoms and manifest the ability to do something effective about them.

Talking to the elderly, the hard of hearing and the elderly frail

Special care is needed from the young professional talking to the elderly and elderly frail. Cultures vary but in modern Britain age is frequently denigrated and old people are no longer valued. Young professionals therefore have a special duty to approach the elderly with respect and dignity. There is an extra need for these encounters to reinforce the self-worth of an elderly person. Autonomy (self-determination) is a global objective of both health and social services. In dealing with the elderly it is a principal objective to maintain the autonomy of older persons. Most health professionals, however, when questioned on attitudes to old age were found to have a negative perspective on ageing, regarding it as an irreversible process of decline and the elderly as being slow and difficult (Coe 1967). Many nurses also express an unwillingness to work with the elderly (Seer 1986).

Young professionals should therefore approach the elderly with the dignity and respect which is their due. Use a dignified style of address 'Good morning Mrs Brown' not 'Hi Gladys' unless you are invited by the patient to do otherwise. Demonstrate a polite demeanour with attentiveness to the patient's concerns. The approach should be relatively formal, straightforward and with direct eye contact. You may need to identify yourself more than once during the consultation and it is important to try and obtain the elderly patient's undivided attention and to eliminate distractions from noise and physical discomfort. Seat the patient close to you and face-to-face in a good light so that the patient can both read your lips and hear your voice. Elderly people lay great store by regular eye contact and this is reassuring as an affirmation of your interest and concern.

Barriers to communication with the elderly

Potential barriers to good communication with the elderly are legion. They may be cognitive, behavioural or physical in nature. Obvious physical problems such as failing eyesight and deafness can prevent the elderly patient from both hearing your voice and reading your lips. Elderly people, however, tend to be sensitive to non-verbal communication and will respond quickly to both positive and negative cues in your behaviour (Grimley Evans 2000). They are frequently socially isolated and as a result lose the skills of normal social interchange. They may be lonely and out of the habit of conversation. The elderly often have low self-esteem, which is a handicap in projecting their needs and wishes. Problems with memory may interfere with the retention of information and with their ability to process rationally the information they do retain. Often old people have numerous ailments and frequently take large numbers of different forms of medication. The complexity of their symptomatology and polypharmacy can make clear communication difficult. Bereavement especially with loss of a supportive spouse or close friend further undermines an old person's self-confidence and deprives them of social support. Establishing relationships with others after bereavement can be difficult especially when a health professional is very much younger.

Elderly people may have difficulty in conversations involving more than two people. Hearing difficulties and reaction time can make it difficult to follow speech from more than one angle. Participation is difficult for an older person when they are not addressed directly in conversation.

Older patients are often accompanied to the consultation by their spouse or offspring. There is a temptation as a result to deal directly with the relative rather than the patient. It may be much easier to communicate with a younger family member but this is demeaning to the older person who is your patient. Acting as if the patient is not there, or not the person of importance, diminishes their self-worth.

Barriers to communication with the elderly

1. Loss of hearing
2. Deteriorating sight
3. Social isolation
4. Low self-esteem
5. Problems with memory
6. Complexity of medical condition
7. Loss of spouse and friends
8. Group conversations

Hearing loss

Comprehending speech is a complex business comprising hearing, seeing, remembering and understanding. Shouting or talking loudly increases the projection of vowels over consonants and leads to jarring of sound appreciation (see below). Shouting is therefore poignantly inappropriate when trying to communicate with the elderly, many of whom are hard of hearing.

When elderly people are losing acuity of hearing their own speech may become monotonous and this can easily be misinterpreted as apathy or depression.

Clues to hearing difficulty are a puzzled expression, a shy smile, an inclination of the head, a hand raised behind the ear, or frequent nods and tentative answers.

Hearing in old age may be adversely affected by childhood middle ear disease, which was common at the time when the current older generation were children. Chronically scarred or perforated ear drums lead to hearing loss. A lifetimes working exposure to noise can also damage hearing as can degenerative changes occurring with advancing years. Visual impairment further impedes the ability to lip read and thus follow conversations: 'I can't hear you doctor. I need my spectacles!'

Pathological changes in the temporal cortex can have an adverse effect on the hearing process. The speed and efficiency of signal processing in the temporal lobe is adversely affected by pathological changes in that part of the brain. These are commonly associated with cerebrovascular disease in old age and especially Alzheimer's disease in which the temporal lobe is among the earliest parts of the brain to be affected. A test for hearing difficulty can be carried out quite simply by whispering a two-digit number about 10 cm from each ear, e.g. 'twenty seven'.

You can do a great service to the elderly patient with hearing loss if you help them to show others how to help. Tell them to ask others to speak slowly and clearly but not to raise their voice.

When the elderly are in hospital nursing staff form an essential link between patients and the outside world. The elderly are often alone and bored and easily lose touch with external events. Older patients are especially particular about roommates and the proximity of other patients as well as the noise level in the ward from TV and radio, and attention to these details can minimize distress.

Communication strategies for the elderly

When speaking to older patients it is essential to speak slowly with a low but resonant voice, which is calm, reassuring, and projects a sense of control. Older people lose the ability to register high-pitched sound and communication is improved in a quiet non-reverberant room. Detecting consonants is crucial to understanding. Vowels sounds tend to be of longer duration and lower frequency but are harder to distinguish. If you consider written as opposed to vocal speech it is evident that confining writing to vowels alone does not make for easy reading. For example, a sentence conveyed by vowels only written 'o ae ou' has little meaning. However, the same sentence written with consonants 'hw r y' is much easier to interpret as 'how are you?' Paradoxically, longer words are easier to understand. They probably contain more consonants and are more readily identifiable. Words such as spectacles or umbrella are easier to comprehend than a short word such as hat. One simple tip is to use your stetho-scope in reverse to help your patient follow what you are saying.

A reversed stethoscope can help a deaf patient hear your question.

Speed of speech is critical to intelligibility. Although foreign languages, for example, are not in fact spoken faster than English we all need more time to process the unfamiliar signal (Isaacs 1992).

Elderly patients do not respond well to an authoritarian approach, which can be self-defeating (Svarstad 1986). A domineering approach leads to concealment on the part of the older patient with consequent loss of important information. Elderly patients are more often non-compliant than younger people. They often think that they do not actually need the treatment given or prefer to stop treatment as an assertion of independence. The demonstration of empathy and sympathy is much more likely to produce compliance.

In view of the fact that the elderly often have multiple ailments and many medications, clarity is essential in discussing their medical welfare. Clearly written lists can be invaluable. The long-term course of chronic illness can in fact foster scepticism in the aged patient about the pointlessness of medical care and eventually promote disenchantment with the doctor–patient relationship (Maddox 1987).

In talking to the elderly who have deterioration in cognitive ability it is important to allow time for responses. The patient may need time to process and understand your question and to respond appropriately. It is wise to use familiar terms in common usage among the older generation such as wireless for radio and cardigan for sweater. If what the patient says to you does not seem to make much sense it is helpful to seek clue words and repeat these to evoke a feeling of being connected. Do not agree with what you don't understand and do not pretend to understand something, which is unintelligible. Make choices simple.

If you are giving instructions try to break down tasks into one step at a time. It is difficult for the elderly to retain a complex series of instructions. Remember also that touch is important. Many old people have very little physical contact in their lives and it is immensely reassuring and comforting when a health professional places an arm around them for a moment or holds their hand.

Remember too that the elderly have led lengthy and often very interesting lives. Their long life span connects us to our past. Many old people are a valuable source of common sense and wisdom, not to mention a rich vein of humour!

Talking to the bereaved

People in Britain, and health professionals are no exception, are hesitant to talk to people who have been recently bereaved. When death occurs in hospital there may be an assumption that the family would prefer to grieve in peace but in fact this is rarely true. In the immediate aftermath of death, relatives find great comfort in talking to staff who have looked after their loved one and it can be very important to have an opportunity to ask questions about the medical or nursing care before the patient died and about events surrounding death. Medical and nursing staff, however, often do not feel comfortable answering these questions and may feel guilty that they have not saved the person who has died. It is understandable that staff members would rather get away and turn their attention to patients who still need their help. Because staff can no longer make things better for this patient they tend to avoid approaching the family. However, it is of fundamental importance to a healthy grieving process that the loss should be acknowledged.

Try to talk about the dead person in a natural inclusive way and to offer understanding and sympathy. After a death relatives react differently. Most people are numb and in shock, some react with initial disbelief:

'I can't believe it.'

'Are you sure you mean my husband?'

'Surely there is some mistake?'

It is especially important when death has been sudden and unexpected that this fact is recognized. It helps enormously to go through the course of events and to help the relatives acknowledge, accept and talk through the reality of death.

Guilt reactions are common: 'I wish I had stopped him driving when he was tired.' 'I wish I had taken her to the doctor sooner.'

Staff frequently fear that they will be blamed for the patient's death and are fearful of relatives' anger. People do manifest grief by angry behaviour but this is anger aimed at the world rather than at you. It can take courage to speak to the bereaved when powerful emotions easily rise to the surface. It is important to realize that none of this anger is personal. It is unwise to answer back or counter anger with anger. It is wiser to say something like 'I can see you're angry and things are difficult for you'. To survive the attack of someone's rage is part of the doctor and nurses professional job.

When death is sudden it can be very helpful to show the relatives the body of the deceased. Although this may be painful at the time it is helpful to the grieving process in the long run. Be ready to support the bereaved, but be prepared also to give them privacy with the deceased if they request it. Sudden death is understandably traumatic and the sense of unreality and consequent numbness is stronger if death is sudden. The grieving process also tends to be longer than if the death was expected.

When there has been a lengthy deterioration there is more time for a family to prepare emotionally for the death itself. This adjustment, which is described as anticipatory grieving, helps the process of coming to terms with death when this finally occurs.

When talking to relatives after a patient's death mention the death certificate and explain what diagnosis is given. Questions, which worry families at such a moment, can cause long-term distress and depression if not addressed at the time when the information is readily available. Uncertainties linger terribly making adjustment to loss especially difficult and prolonged (Marrow 1996).

The processes of grieving are particularly well described by Kubler Ross (1993) and Worden (1982).

Practical tips

1. Do not avoid bereaved relatives.
2. Acknowledge their loss. Talk through events prior to and during the dying process.
3. Help relatives understand and acknowledge.
4. Talk about the dead person in a natural and inclusive way.
5. Ensure that relatives understand the statements made on the death certificate.

References

Coe, R.N. (1967). Professional prospective on the aged. *Gerontologist*, (7), 114–19.

Fields, S.D. (1991). History taking in the elderly: obtaining useful information. *Geriatrics*, 46(8), 26–35.

Grimley Evans, J. (ed.) (2000). *Oxford Textbook of Geriatric Medicine*. Oxford: Oxford University Press.

Intrieri, R.C., Kelly, J.A., Brown, M.M., Castilla, C. (1993). Improving medical students attitudes toward and skills with the elderly. *Gerontologist*, 33(3), 373–8.

Isaacs, B. (ed.) (1992). *The Challenge of Geriatric Medicine*. Oxford: Oxford University Press.

Kubler Ross, E. (1993). *On Death and Dying*. Routledge.

Maddox, G.L. (ed.) (1987). *The Encyclopedia of Aging*. New York: Springer.

Marrow, J. (1996). Developing communication skills in medicine; Telling relatives that a family member has died suddenly. *Postgraduate Medical Journal*, 72, 413–18.

Morse, J.M., Intrieri, R.C. (1997). 'Talk to me.' Patient communication in a long-term care facility. *Journal of Psychosocial Nursing & Mental Health Services*, 35(5), 34–9.

Parr Sally, Cancer Counsellor, 2003 personal communication.

Seers, C. (1986). Talking to the elderly and its relevance to care. *Nursing Times* 8 January.

Teenage Cancer Trust Secretariat, London 2003.

Worden, J.W. (1982). *Grief Counselling and Grief Therapy: a handbook for the mental health practitioner*. New York: Springer.

Chapter 10

Difficult practical circumstances

Elisabeth Macdonald

Summary

This chapter identifies some of the practical issues involved in talking to patients over the telephone, via an interpreter or recording the conversation on audiotape. Some difficult issues raised in dealing with close or collusive relatives are addressed.

Telephone consultations

It can be very difficult to discuss serious health issues over the telephone. However, the telephone and especially the mobile phone are now fundamental to the way we live our lives and the natural way for most of us to communicate. Communication is made easier if the phone call involves a patient or family member with whom you are familiar. If you know the patient well it is relatively easy to tune into their responses and to judge what it is safe to discuss and what would be better discussed face to face. On the whole it is much better to deliver serious news when you have the patient with you. First, you can ensure by reading their facial expression and body language that they have understood the information you are seeking to communicate, and secondly, it is possible for you to respond much more appropriately to any emotional reaction that the patient may experience. It is then possible to spend more time with a distressed patient and to ensure that they are not left alone once your conversation has ended. If a patient receives unexpected and unpleasant news while at home there may be many hours, for example, before their spouse returns home to give moral support. If a patient is home alone or out at work there may be no one with whom to share the burden of bad news and it is much more difficult to keep natural anxiety in proportion when there is no one with whom to discuss it. With the advent of the mobile phone someone receiving a call may find himself or herself in a very inappropriate situation to listen to medical information or discuss confidential matters. They may, however, fear that the doctor will ring off and the opportunity be lost if they don't accept the call. When making a phone call to a patient or relative it is therefore important to check that the time and place of the call are convenient and private:

'Have I caught you at a good or a bad moment?'

'Shall I call back later?'

'Would you prefer to call me back on this number?'

If there is really no alternative to delivering bad news by telephone then it is worth ringing the patient to ask when would be a convenient time for you to call back with news 'when it is available', establishing when there will be moral support available for the patient. In the event of serious conversations by telephone it is also vital for the patient to know how to get back to you with further queries and therefore essential to leave a return phone number and details of your availability (after a clinic or operating session, for example).

A better alternative if at all practicable is to ask the patient to come in and see you in your usual consultation environment, whether the clinic, practice or ward and arrange to sit down together to discuss the new developments in the clinical situation. Patients will guess that the news is bad or at least complicated and will have time to prepare. A period of apprehension is less distressing than a poorly managed telephone conversation that fails to provide the right level of empathy, information and explanation.

Telephone calls that fall more in the category of counselling conversations are a very different matter. It can be immensely helpful for a patient to have the opportunity to talk to a doctor or nurse with whom they are already familiar while in the security of his or her own environment. Patients are then often more relaxed and able to think more clearly and formulate the questions that they really need answered. It can underline the normality of the relationship when a doctor bothers to call by phone and finds the time to spend in discussion.

Consultation through an interpreter

When there are severe language difficulties it can be essential to use the services of an interpreter to facilitate communication with the patient or family. Wherever possible it is wise to use professional independent interpreters who have no ulterior motives or hidden agenda. Nor in principle do they have any emotional involvement that can complicate the translation of certain issues.

Family members on the other hand, when translating for a relative, often with the best of intentions, may seek to cloud or conceal bad news in an attempt to protect their family members. Some families deliberately choose to consult a doctor who does not speak their own language in order that the family can control the flow of information to the patient. For example, if a patient has been diagnosed with malignant disease some families prefer to conceal this diagnosis from a patient especially when elderly. The family may believe that the patient will be so distressed by the diagnosis that he or she will simply give up and refuse treatment. Cultural differences in approach to serious illness need sensitive handling and these issues are further covered in Chapter 12.

A major difficulty in working through interpreters is that the doctor simply does not know how accurately her words are being translated or even whether accurate words exist in translation. One can often tell from the patient's reaction whether the translation is roughly correct but neither the patient nor the doctor can truly control the accuracy of the exchange. Confidential issues that may be fundamental to the health problem can simply be withheld or not translated.

Further problems can arise between generations. Some older immigrant members of our community have not either by choice or opportunity learnt English and may bring with them to the consultation a junior member of the family who is more likely to speak the language. Previously confidential issues may emerge to the distress both of the relative and the patient. Health issues can be discussed that may have implications for the interpreter too. Information about disease, which is communicated genetically or by infection of close contacts, may place a heavy burden on the family translator. The responsibility of some privileged knowledge may be far greater than the interpreter had contemplated.

The generation gap can also cause considerable problems with embarrassment over intimate questioning. It is clearly inappropriate to discuss, for example, the exact details of gynaecological symptoms for an elderly lady whose consultation is being interpreted by her grandson. This type of conversation is much better conducted through an independent interpreter. However, there are communities from many parts of the world speaking rare languages for whom interpretation outside their own community poses great difficulty.

The other major issue in working through interpreters is that of confidentiality. Professional interpreters employed by hospitals are in theory required to conform to a professional undertaking to preserve confidentiality and this in theory forms part of the contract of all health-care workers. Interpreters from the patient's own social group should be instructed at the outset that a medical consultation is privileged and that the information discussed is confidential.

Practical tips: conducting consultations through an interpreter

When a patient and family arrive at a consultation with an interpreter it is sensible to establish from the outset who speaks English and who does not. Separately it is wise to establish who understands English, although they may not be able to speak the language. Many newcomers pick up a lot of English, for example from television, although they cannot find the words to speak themselves. It is then worth explaining briefly to an interpreter what you understand their role to mean. You expect them to translate accurately as far as possible without either summarizing or elaborating on your words. The general duty of confidentiality should be mentioned with the expectation that secrets will be preserved within the confines of the consultation.

When using an interpreter it is essential to address your questions and statements directly to the patient rather than to the interpreter. It is natural to look at and speak to the person who understands but it is important to show that you are concentrating on the patient and not on their interpreter. It is helpful to keep your sentences short, your terminology simple and non-medical and your approach warm and patient. Treat the interpreter as an 'assistant' and remember to thank them specifically for their help.

Because of language difficulties it may not be possible to cover in one consultation all the ground that you would normally be able to encompass in a single visit with an English speaking patient. A return visit may need to scheduled. However, the difficulty of bringing the interpreter, the patient and doctor together at the same time often leads unfortunately to increased brevity in an attempt to cover all the salient issues in a single interview. Although this is undesirable, it may be the lesser of two evils.

Written information in the patient's mother tongue or local dialect can be enormously helpful, enabling the patient to come to terms with medical information in their own way and helping them prepare for a further consultation when necessary.

It is also wise to be aware that many interpreters feel that they are not only the patient's spokesman but also their advocate. Many interpreters do become emotionally involved with families for whom they translate frequently and this can be difficult both for the interpreter and the doctor. They may provide information that they think will influence the doctor favourably, for example to admit a patient to hospital, rather than that which is a true reflection of the facts. On the other hand distressing matters may be downplayed in either direction in the interpreter's effort to protect themselves from exposure to sadness and pain. Good interpreters, however, are an invaluable source of cultural information and can steer you away from an unwitting cultural indiscretion if you can successfully create a good working relationship.

Practical tips: consultations through an interpreter

1. Establish who speaks English
2. Establish who understands English
3. State that medical confidentiality applies
4. Address yourself to the patient directly and not to the interpreter
5. Include the interpreter appropriately as a colleague
6. Thank the interpreter on conclusion for his or her assistance

Recording consultations on audiotape

Many patients have expressed dissatisfaction with the amount of information given to them by their doctors. One explanation given is shortness of time on the part of the doctor leading to omission of information that the patient considers important but the doctor does not. Poor communication skills possessed by doctors may also contribute to this dissatisfaction. Some doctors on the other hand, in certain circumstances, deliberately withhold information in order to reduce the likelihood of information overload or distress on the part of the patient. A further explanation may be that patients hearing unpleasant news tend to forget later information or repress this knowledge especially when they have been shocked or emotionally disturbed by 'bad news' in the early part of an interview.

A number of suggestions have been made to improve the transfer of information from doctor to patient. The presence of a relative or friend not only acts as an emotional support but also facilitates the communication of information. Being less emotionally involved than the patient with the impact of the information given, a friend or relative often recalls more of the interview in later discussions.

An alternative method of improving the communication of information is the use of informative leaflets, written information or video recordings. Many of these are extremely useful and provide fairly accurate material in a clear, easily understandable manner. They can, however, also be too general for individual patients and may even include information that is inappropriate or misleading for the particular patient (Hogbin 1989).

One way to circumvent this problem and to ensure that the information that is given is wholly appropriate and specifically designed to meet the individual patient's needs is to provide an audiotape of the patient's actual consultation with the doctor. On the face of it the taping of important conversations for the patient to play back at a later date, both for themselves and their relatives, would seem an entirely sensible and positive procedure. However, some drawbacks have been identified and on the whole doctors have not viewed this suggestion favourably.

Advantages of taping consultations

Doctors whose consultations 'delivering bad news' have been recorded became more aware of the need to do this properly. The fact of recording the interview also gave the bad news consultation a rather higher profile and doctors volunteer that this made them consciously attach even more importance to the consultation than they had done previously (Hogbin 1989).

Doctors on the whole, however, do not seem to view the taping of conversations with much enthusiasm. Although it is evident that patients often do not take in all that they are told during a consultation and that an audiotape recording offers the opportunity to revisit this information, some doctors find that the tape recorder 'casts a shadow' over the consultation. An awareness of the recorder running can cramp the style of both doctor and patient and this will not enhance communication. Some doctors, while happy to cooperate with a patient who brings in a tape recorder, will not volunteer this facility themselves (R. Rubens, ICRF Professor of Medical Oncology, personal communication, 2000). Although the use of tapes has been advocated to enhance physician/patient communication since 1977 (Butt 1977) few doctors have incorporated tape recording into their practice (McConnell *et al.* 1999). In response to surveys on the subject doctors who are not enthusiastic about providing consultation audiotapes cite such issues as patient confidentiality and medico-legal concerns as reasons for their reluctance (Tattersall and Butow 2002).

Patients on the other hand view the use of tapes during important consultations with much greater enthusiasm. Patients on the whole have found their tape recordings extremely helpful for a variety of different reasons (Hogbin 1989). Not only do the majority of patients listen to them several times themselves but also most people play them to various other family members and friends. This can be especially helpful when families are geographically widespread as tapes can be easily sent in the post. Another advantage is that lay people often have problems recalling medical terminology or the names of procedures about which they have little previous knowledge and these can be checked again from the tape. Doctors tend to overestimate the ability of patients to understand even fairly simple medical terms and this difficulty is compounded further when a patient is emotionally distressed (Samora *et al.* 1961; Segall and Roberts 1980). If phrases can be replayed, perhaps to the family doctor, then unfamiliar terms and areas of confusion can be clarified.

One major and perhaps unexpected benefit of tape recording difficult conversations is the assistance it gives the patient in sharing bad news or describing a complicated situation to spouse or family. Just as doctors find it difficult to break bad news to patients, or to explain difficult concepts, so patients themselves often find the prospect of telling their loved ones that they have a serious illness extremely distressing. Many patients have voiced the view that the primary value of the tapes was their usefulness in giving accurate information to the family (Hogbin 1989). In addition, hearing the calm and reasoned discussion that took place, can be reassuring not only to the family, but can also calm the patient during times of panic and despair. In other words the tenor of the discussion can continue to reassure and help to keep things in perspective.

Disadvantages of taping conversations

One major disadvantage from the patient's point of view must, however, be borne in mind. When studying the efficacy of audiotapes in promoting psychological well-being in cancer patients McHugh *et al.* (1995) noted that those patients who had a poor prognosis were specifically disadvantaged by access to the tape. Maguire and Pitceathly (2002) have also voiced this reservation: 'If you have to give the patient a poor prognosis providing an audiotape may hinder psychological adjustment.' It is easy to imagine the despair engendered by sitting alone listening again and again to a doom-laden forecast and contemplating one's own extinction. When the outlook is dire it is much kinder to avoid taping the consultation and to concentrate on positive aspects such as symptom control and to see the patient regularly if possible.

One further potential disadvantage is probably overstressed. Some doctors feel that litigious patients may try to use the tape recording as proof of negligence in that, for example, too little or inaccurate information was provided. However, as long as the doctor behaves reasonably, such a record is more likely to provide an incontrovertible defence to the claim.

On the whole most research in this area draws positive conclusions in favour of the use of tapes. Clear evidence supports the contention that there is improvement in factual retention, although evidence is so far lacking that there is reduction in psychological distress using this approach.

Conversations with spouse or partner

When talking to a spouse or partner it is wise to take your cue from the patient. One cannot presume conventional relationships and there is wide variation in the trust that exists between partners. The balance of power between individuals may not be self-evident and on public occasions such as hospital visits partners may put a brave face on things for the sake of appearances. It is wise to ask the patient with whom, if anyone, he or she would like you to share information. The 'legitimate' husband or wife may not in fact be the patient's confidante at all!

Surprises can even be comical. One dear lady on being reassured that her husband's prognosis was not as bad as first thought was heard to exclaim, 'Oh no! I've 'ad 50 years of 'ell with that man!'

Collusive relatives

Although honesty in medical matters as between staff, patients and relatives is now the norm, there still exist families from many cultures who seek to protect family members from information that they judge is likely to cause undue distress. These families may try to recruit your support in misleading a patient about, for example, the seriousness of a diagnosis. Part of the motivation often stems from the relatives' own dread of witnessing the distress of a loved one as well as the desire to spare the patient anxiety.

In view of your clear ethical duty to respect your patient's autonomy and right to know the truth this invitation needs to be gently but firmly resisted. This kind of conspiracy instead of increasing the patient's well-being, on the contrary tends to leave the patient feeling uneasy and excluded, aware that important information is being withheld.

How can this request for collusive behaviour be resisted?

When you encounter a collusive relative start by asking them why they don't want to tell the patient the truth: 'Could you tell me why you want to keep the truth from your wife and why you don't want the doctors to speak to her either?'

The husband will probably give the sort of explanation outlined above. Contradicting this view directly is unlikely to be helpful. Instead work at developing an otherwise trusting relationship and explore how he feels at misleading his wife: 'How does it make you feel knowing you are not being honest with your wife?'

You will probably find that it is the source of great tension and despondency. Explore also how this pretence is affecting his relationship with his wife. You will probably find that there is increasing distance and tension here also:

'How are things between you and your wife these days?'

'Do you feel as close as usual?'

'Or are there some problems?'

Once these problems are acknowledged you can contrast this continuing unhappiness with the short-term distress you may encounter by being honest. Facing the truth together is usually followed by increased closeness and the comfort and satisfaction of sharing reactions, thoughts and plans.

Offer to talk to the patient in the presence of the wife or husband so that both parties hear the same information and can discuss it together when ready. Acknowledge that both sides want to do the best for each other but are in the end hurting rather than helping the other.

Practical tips to deal with collusion

1. Resist the invitation to collude with misinformation.
2. Explore the effect of collusion on the relative's psychological comfort.
3. Explore the effect on the relationship.
4. Offer to talk things through with both parties together.

References

Butt, H.R. (1977). A method for better physician-patient communication. *Annals of Internal Medicine*, **86**, 478–80.

Hogbin, B. (1989). Getting it taped: the 'bad news' consultation with cancer patients. *British Journal of Hospital Medicine*, **42**, 330–3.

Maguire, P., Pitceathly, C. (2002). Key communication skills and how to acquire them. *British Medical Journal*, **325**(7366), 697–700.

McConnell, D., Butow, P.N., Tattersall, M.H. (1999). Audio-tapes and letters to patients; the practice and views of oncologists, surgeons and general practitioners. *British Journal of Cancer*, **79**(11–12), 1782–8.

McHugh, P., Lewis, S., Ford, S., Newlands, E., Rustin, G., Coombes, C., Smith, D., O'Reilly, S., Fallowfield, L. (1995). The efficacy of audiotapes in promoting psychological well-being in cancer patients: a randomised controlled trial. *British Journal of Cancer*, **71**(2), 388–92.

Samora, J., Saunders, L., Larson, M. (1961). Medical vocabulary knowledge among hospital patients. *Journal of Health and Human Behavior*, **2**, 83–9.

Segall, A., Roberts, L.W. (1980). A comparative analysis of physician estimates and levels of medical knowledge among patients. *Sociology of Health and Illness*, **2**, 317–34.

Tattersall, M.H., Butow, P.N. (2002). Consultation audiotapes; An underused cancer patient information aid and clinical research tool. *Lancet Oncology*, **3**(7), 431–7.

Chapter 11

Communication in a multiprofessional setting

Cathy Heaven

Summary

The chapter is written in three parts. First, it will look at how and why doctors' conversations with patients may differ from those of other colleagues. Secondly, it will focus on how working with colleagues may help make difficult conversations easier, through using other expertise, and also through sharing different perspectives. The third section looks at how difficult conversations with colleagues, for example disagreements, may be managed more effectively, and how communication within teams can be improved.

Differences in conversations

Doctors' conversations with patients and relatives may differ from those of their professional colleagues for a number of reasons. The most obvious reason is that each group of professionals has a different area of interest and expertise. Thus each professional will have a slightly different focus depending on training, interest and overall goal. For example, a doctor with a high degree of training in anatomy, physiology and pathophysiology, who wishes to talk to a patient so that he or she can establish the chronology of events and a detailed picture of the illness, with a view to forming a diagnosis and treatment plan, is bound to pick up and focus on different cues to a nurse. The nurse, who is trained to a lesser level in anatomy, physiology and pathophysiology, will wish to establish the impact of the illness on the patient and family in a holistic sense so as to identify care needs and formulate a care plan. While the two interviews will inevitably overlap, the difference in focus, and the sensitivity to different types of cues and problems will mean that the two conversations will also in the end appear different, and will lead to different plans of action (Crow *et al.* 1995; Bornstein and Emler 2001).

Attention to different cues, because of differing cognitive processes is discussed at length by Crow *et al.* (1995). Crow *et al.* argue that context specific knowledge is developed through experience and forms the basis of expertise. The presence of specific expertise has been established for doctors, nurses, physicists, bridge players and others, and enables the individual to limit the amount of information needed through filtering out irrelevant material and linking up relevant material. Thus in a medical assessment a doctor will, through expertise, attach different meaning to information gathered, filter out different information and make different links between pieces of information, compared to other colleagues.

Across the spectrum of professional conversations some topics are often associated with certain professionals, e.g. the doctor with discussions about diagnosis, trials and treatment, whereas other areas, e.g. discharge planning or emotional support are more commonly considered the domain of other professional groups, such as nurses, occupational therapists, social workers, psychologists or chaplains. Making these types of generalizations may help us to understand why conversations in health care may differ, but it is vital that it does not lead to the belief that certain domains are, or are not, within the remit of certain health professionals. Unfortunately, there is evidence that this type of 'pigeon holing' has been partially responsible for breakdown in communication. The belief that 'it is not my role to discuss such things' has been found to contribute to the poor identification of patient concerns (Heaven and Maguire 1997), and also to health-care professionals' blocking of patient cues (Maguire 1985).

Effective communication, as described by those who have spent many years researching the field, is described as that which involves eliciting and responding to problems, concerns or worries in all areas (Maguire 1999; Dowsett *et al.* 2000; Fallowfield *et al.* 2002). It has been shown that patients who don't get the chance to disclose all their concerns (whether physical, or emotional) are more anxious after consultations (Macleod 1991) more dissatisfied (Korsch and Negrete 1972) and more likely to complain (Ley 1982). It is important to add here that listening to a patient's concerns, is not the same as dealing with all the concerns. It is often the case that many of the concerns expressed need no action or a simple acknowledgement, or a referral to a more appropriate person. For the patient it is the opportunity to express the concerns and the fact that they feel the doctor has a clear understanding of them, which appears to be of benefit (Maguire 1985; Pennebaker 1993).

A final reason that medical and other health-care conversations differ is the influence of the patients and/or relatives themselves. Studies looking at disclosure have shown that patients not only withhold information from their medical carers (Cole-Kelly 1992) but also disclose different things to different people, so influencing the course of the conversation.

A variety of different reasons have been documented for this. A study of hospice patients' disclosure patterns revealed that the patients withheld up to 60% of the concerns they were experiencing. Content analysis demonstrated that patients were revealing only certain types of concerns suggesting that they believed that certain professionals were only interested in certain types of issues. This phenomenon has also been reported elsewhere (Maguire 1985; Higginson and McCarthy 1993). Other documented reasons for withholding information from medical carers include fear, for example fear of criticism for those such as smokers whose life-styles could have contributed to the illness, fear of being seen as complaining, for example, about side-effects, or fear of being told some bad news if questions are asked (Maguire 1985; Parker and Hopwood 2000). Patients also fear losing composure, and so avoid key issues, or fear overburdening the doctor, whom often they can see is busy and tired.

Presumptions that certain problems are inevitable and must be put up with or that a problem cannot be alleviated also lead to non-disclosure to the doctor. Awareness of just how busy wards and clinics are is a considerable factor, as many patients perceive that doctors do not have enough time to go into all their worries. They therefore prioritize worries by what they think the doctors want to hear about, falling into the trap of believing that certain doctors are only interested in certain types of problems or concerns (Heaven and Maguire 1997; Anderson *et al.* 2001).

Other factors that inhibit patients disclosing to doctors include lack of privacy from people overhearing what is being said, especially in a ward environment, or a lack of space away from key individuals in front of whom that patient or relative may not wish to discuss certain fears, e.g. spouses, children, etc. Many health professionals do not consider the impact of the presence of a family member on an interview. Indeed in palliative care, professionals positively encourage the carer to be present when interviewing the patient (Heaven 2001); however, this may lead to many concerns being withheld, as patients actively protect their relatives (Pistrang and Barker 1992).

For all these reasons, when interviewing the same patient each nurse or doctor will exit a conversation with a different, but accurate view of the situation. Without discussion each is only privy to one view, or one side of the story. It is therefore a poor clinician who does not recognize the importance of discussing cases with colleagues and actively seeking colleagues' views of the situation, and who does not realize the value of using other professionals to help manage the many complex and difficult situations that can arise in health care.

Working with colleagues

Working nurses: teamwork and changing roles

Close working relationships between doctors and their nursing colleagues have developed differently in various parts of medicine. In many specialities, e.g. cancer care, close working relationships based on mutual respect and autonomy can be seen, and the resultant advantages are reported. These include enhanced patient care (Bredin *et al.* 1999), broader range of services offered (Glajchen *et al.* 1995), more time to focus on areas of speciality (Thompson 1995), greater job satisfaction (Jenkins *et al.* 2001), and enhanced source of support to all those involved (Oberle and Hughes 2001).

However, development and changes in roles, for example nurses taking the lead in what were traditionally medical areas, such as bone marrow biopsies, running follow-up clinics or prescribing certain drugs, has led to uncomfortable and difficult periods of change. Shifts in traditional domains of knowledge and responsibility, and blurring of role boundaries has led to resentment and bad feeling among medical and nursing professionals alike, and this has manifested itself in rivalry and at times open hostility. However, it is vital that all health-care professionals recognize that the loser in this situation is the patient (Madge and Khair 2000).

Interpersonal communication is at the heart of sorting out the difficulties that both the changes in role and the traditional differences in approach have created. This chapter has been written with the hope of creating greater understanding of the value of the differences in approach, and also to look at ways in which junior doctors may use their colleagues, nursing and others, to help them manage difficult situations.

Involving colleagues in difficult conversations

Taking a colleague with you into a difficult interview is not only a good idea, but is advocated at all levels (Girghis and Sanson-Fisher 1995; Mager and Andryowski 2002). The old adage, 'two heads are better than one' couldn't be more pertinent than when dealing with a group of relatives, an angry complaining patient, or a couple who have differing views on treatment.

Joint interviewing has benefits for all involved. For patients, repetition of separate assessment visits is avoided, cues are more likely to be picked up, and if a person has already spoken to the colleague, there is the potential for them to feel more empowered to be clearer about difficulties. For the doctor there is the benefit of additional insights through listening to the approach of a colleague, recognizing how cues may be missed, much needed support when a conversation has been particularly harrowing, and the opportunity for feedback on performance, if the doctor is brave enough to ask for it. Finally, for the colleague there is a greater insight into what actually happened, and how the patients or relative behaved when faced with their difficulties. This can often lead to greater empathy and understanding toward the doctor, as well as greater team cohesion and support. The final advantage for both colleague and doctor is the reduction of reliance on third party reporting of conversations, or on annotations in the notes.

Working in tandem with colleagues is not always straight forward, especially on the first occasion. Discussion prior to the visit, as to format and who is taking the lead, can reduce many of the practical difficulties.

Talking to colleagues before visits

It is not always possible to arrange joint visits with colleagues, in this situation a discussion prior to a consultation can provide a forum for sharing of knowledge and understanding of the situation, as well as helping identify key areas that need addressing with the patient. Many nurses, especially specialist nurses, are in a position to gain insights into the impact of any illness and its treatment on the whole family situation, partly because they have the opportunity to meet with and spend more time with the patient and with the family, and partly, as already discussed, because this is a more direct part of their role. This puts many nurses in the unique position of being able to follow-up on patients and their partners, both in the hospital and in the community, and helps them gain a greater understanding of what has been assimilated from medical consultations, and also any resultant hopes, fears and needs. Specialist nurses are often the key in directing patients back to clinic to get specific questions answered, or to discuss specific options. In the ward environment because of the physical nature of their caring role, nurses have the opportunity to spend time with patients in a relaxed informal situation. During these informal settings conversations often happen which give great insights into the patient's thinking. Concerns and fears are expressed that may be withheld in a more formal interview situation, as a sort of testing ground to see if problems are significant, (Macleod-Clarke 1983; Maguire 1985; Heaven and Maguire 1998).

Reviewing these things with a colleague, prior to an interview will provide clarity for the doctor in understanding whether there is a specific need to be addressed, and will also help in anticipating potentially difficult areas that may be encountered. It will also give an insight into factors normally not assessed in a medical follow-up, but which could have a tremendous impact on such things as compliance, effectiveness and side-effects.

Referring patients to colleagues

There are numerous specialist professions working within the health-care system all of whom have specialist knowledge in their own particular area. The system of referral between medical colleagues for specialist opinion is a normal part of patient care, as is referral to some non-medical specialities, e.g. physiotherapy. Other specialist professionals, e.g. occupational therapists, dieticians, clinical psychologists, chaplains, social workers, etc.; are less commonly involved in medical care, and therefore many doctors are less familiar with their role and the exact expertise they can offer. Using colleagues to give help with difficult situations can be immensely useful, given that, as already discussed, patients will tell different professionals different things.

The system of referral to other colleagues differs between hospitals; for example, some require a medical referral, whereas in other institutions nurses may refer patients. They key to any referral, if it is to be effective, is the patient's awareness of and consent to the process. For example, a patient who has not been informed of a referral to a clinical psychologists may well refuse to talk, or walk out when faced with the situation. Many doctors and nurses express the concern that when informed of the intention to refer, some patients will refuse. While this may be the case, it is important to acknowledge that, not only does the patient have the right to know about a referral, but also that in discussing it the opportunity to talk about the doctor's reasons and the patient's concerns is created, before the time of a busy colleague is wasted.

Communication within a multiprofessional team

Difficult conversations with colleagues

There are many occasions in health care when differences of opinion arise, some of which can lead to difficulties in working relationships between staff, be they from the same discipline or from different professional groupings. While problems within professional groupings can be difficult to deal with, the hierarchical structure of each discipline forms a framework for dealing, or not dealing, with the issues as they arise. Difficulties across professional groups cause more problems, as there is often a less clear hierarchical structure, and different lines of responsibility.

Working with colleagues in multidisciplinary groups can lead to all sorts of difficulties as areas of expertise and roles overlap. There are many things that lead to disagreements about the way forward with care. For example, the efficacy of continuing treatment or about the appropriateness for certain patients of types of treatment; about communication, for example, the level of information being given or the way someone is spoken to; or about the attitude of the professional colleague to either the patient and family or to another colleague. In the past the strongly hierarchical health-care system in which senior medical and nursing staff had immense power meant that decisions and attitudes were never questioned (Menzies 1961; Hammond and Mosley 2002). Changes in the way staff work together in teams and in the way patients are cared for, has led to closer working relationships and greater opportunity for colleagues to see how other teams practice. This has on many occasions provided a great learning opportunity for all those involved. However, on occasions strong differences of opinion arise. Without the opportunity to discuss differences in an adaptive and informative manner these can lead to resentment, and undermine team moral.

The impact of staff conflict is widely acknowledged (Ramirez *et al.* 1996; Wilkinson 1991; Booth *et al.* 1996). Wilkinson (1991) showed that nurses experiencing staff conflict were more likely to distance themselves from patients' emotions, while Booth *et al.* (1996) showed that those who felt supported at work were less likely to block patients. What starts as simple differences of opinion can often lead to major rifts in teams, and causes of great antagonism. Within training workshops health-care professionals are very quick to identify the actions of others that cause them distress (Maguire and Faulkner 1988), and equally quick to realize that if they had been dealt with at an early stage, these issues would not cause the distress currently attributed to them. Learning to deal quickly and efficiently with small differences of opinion, and tackling those difficulties that are causing real problems is therefore not only going to benefit each individual, but will also benefit those patients and families that they care for.

There are a number of difficult conversations we have to undertake with colleagues, but none more so than confronting a colleague's difficult behaviour with the aim of attaining a change, without destroying ones working relationships.

Talking to a colleague about undesirable behaviour

Throughout this section the strategy will be demonstrated using an example, which is set out below.

> The colleague of a doctor is often unrealistically optimistic with patients; telling them they will be fine, when this is either untrue, or very unlikely. The colleague has created a number of problems for the doctor in dealing with patients and families, including, creating confusion and anger by giving contradicting information that results in mixed

messages. Recently, a patient, Mr J, was left very upset and angry. The colleague had told him he would be fine, and the treatment was going well, when the results clearly indicated the contrary. The doctor then, an hour later, had to tell Mr J that the treatment was not working and nothing else could be offered.

Preparation

One of the reasons that talking to a colleague in these types of situations is hard, is because we fear the reaction from our colleague, be it anger, distress or hurt. In many ways telling a colleague something that they are not going to like hearing, is akin to breaking bad news. In much the same way, it is important to prepare for the encounter, being clear about the information you wish to impart, or the evidence of the behaviour that is causing the problems. Secondly, it is important to have a good idea about what you want to get out of the conversation, i.e. are you hoping to achieve a change of behaviour, a plan of action or simply an apology. Within the example given, preparation may include the following:

1. Being clear about the situation with Mr J.
2. What happened.
3. The problems it caused for Mr J, by giving him the mixed messages.
4. Any other examples of similar situations.
5. What is wanted out of the interview.
6. Colleague agrees that being overoptimistic is not always appropriate. That he/she agrees to try to change.

Setting up the time and place

It is vital that you do not confront someone when you are angry, as emotion is likely to take over and the conversation will descend into a row. Therefore, consider when an appropriate time may be, and make an appointment with the colleague to talk about the problem. For example:

Doctor: 'There is something important that I want to talk to you about'

Colleague: 'Oh. OK. What is it?'

Doctor: 'It is to do with one of our patients. It needs about 15 minutes of your time to go through it'.

Colleague: 'Oh right'

Doctor: 'Would after lunch be OK?'

Note how in the initial opening, it is important not to minimize the situation by using the phrase 'want a chat', or by apologizing for needing to talk. The phrase 'something important' also acts like a warning shot, indicating a serious issue. Note also that even though an explanation was invited by the colleague, the situation was not discussed then and there; the whole thing was put on hold until the there was sufficient time and space.

Confronting the situation

The key to addressing any grievance or cause of concern with a colleague is to come to the point quickly, to state the situation as you see it clearly and concisely, say what the problem is, and why. In situations of anxiety and concern about others reactions it is easy to waffle, apologize and understate the concern. This should be avoided, as shown in the example:

Doctor: 'I wanted to talk to you about something that is really concerning me'

Colleague: 'Oh yes'

Doctor: 'It is to do with how we as a team respond to patients fears about how treatment is going'

Colleague: 'Oh right'

Doctor: 'It has come to my attention that on several occasions you have responded to patients by giving a very optimistic view of how their treatment is going, when, in fact, things are not going well at all. I am in the situation of having to give patients very different messages and this has lead to much confusion'

Colleague: 'What do you mean very optimistic . . . I . . . .'

Doctor: 'Perhaps I could give you an example. On Wednesday Mr J asked directly how things were going, I understand from him, that you assured him everything was going fine, and told him he was worrying unnecessarily. An hour later, I had to tell him about the results of his tests, he was devastated'

Colleague: 'I thought it better he did not worry until we had something concrete to tell him . . . .'

Doctor: 'I appreciate that, but you and I both knew that things were going badly. In being so optimistic, you created false hope for Mr J, which then made it much more difficult for him to hear the bad news later. He was very angry about it, in his words he was being "messed around by us." '

In stating the situation it is important to remain factual, not personal; to accept what a colleague says, but not to be deterred from the issue you need to deal with. If a problem is ongoing, have a number of examples ready so that a response to one, does not leave you without any clear argument.

The key to confronting any behaviour is to keep the conversation as neutral as possible. If your colleague is annoyed or affronted by an accusation it is easy for them to disagree with you, and argue about whose point of view may be correct or better. If, however, you can keep the argument patient centred, and put it in terms of the problem caused for the patient, then it avoids things becoming personal, making it much less likely that the conversation will deteriorate into an argument. In the above example it was the reaction of the patient that was put as the reason for the conversation, and not the personal opinion of the doctor.

Moving on to resolution

For the majority of situations the reasons for having these difficult conversations is not to get an apology, but to try to trigger the colleague into changing their behaviour so as to prevent future problems and create a better working environment, for you, your colleagues and most importantly to improve patient care. It is therefore very important to be sensitive to a colleague's acceptance that things may not have been done well, and move on to how they can be improved, without necessarily expecting an apology or admission of wrong-doing.

> *Doctor:* 'The situation with Mr J has now been dealt with and hopefully resolved, but I guess my main reason for talking to you today is to see if we can prevent this type of thing happening again'.
>
> *Colleague:* 'I don't see how we can.'
>
> *Doctor:* 'Well . . . from the patients' points of view . . . it is about not giving mixed messages. Which means not giving unrealistic hope or false expectations'.
>
> *Colleague:* 'But that is really hard—you can't just say, well it doesn't look good Mr J, can you?'
>
> *Doctor:* 'No, but there are things that we can say, which are still honest, but don't get us into the situation of giving false hope, as happened this week'.
>
> *Colleague:* 'Like what?'

Note how the central focus of the conversation continued to be the situation for the patient, and how by using we, instead of you, the doctor made the problem not the colleague but the difficult situation being faced. This enabled the colleague to show that the reason for the behaviour was lack of skills, and thus opened up a potential for training as a possible solution to the situation.

Summary

The overall strategy in addressing this difficult conversation has been first to keep it patient centred, not personal. To break the news clearly and concisely and to stick to the point when distracted, and to move on to identifying a resolution as soon as possible, rather than waiting for some kind of acceptance of wrong doing.

Practical tips: talking to a colleague about undesirable behaviour

- ◆ Choose appropriate time
- ◆ Let anger pass
- ◆ Make appointment with colleague
- ◆ Mention 'something important'
- ◆ Come to the point quickly
- ◆ Be clear and concise
- ◆ Say what the problem is and why
- ◆ Be factual not personal
- ◆ Do not be deterred
- ◆ Have examples ready
- ◆ Keep conversation neutral
- ◆ Keep your arguments patient centred
- ◆ Move rapidly on to a resolution

Improving communication within the multidisciplinary team

Many health professionals report frustration in communicating with colleagues (Maguire and Faulkner 1988; Fallowfield *et al.* 1998), but very little research has been conducted in this area to identify the main factors involved. Many concerns are expressed in communication skills workshop training about lack of communication within teams and slowness of communication between teams and professional groupings, or hospital and community, due to formal referral procedures and traditional reliance on letter writing (Maguire and Faulkner 1988; Fallowfield *et al.* 1998).

A study of 48 nurses showed that much of the written interprofessional reporting was task orientated, focused on medical treatments, and failed to cover psychological and social aspects of care (Dowding 2001). The study also showed that during shift reports nurses recorded less than half the information given or discussed, and recalled less than 27%. There was a clear bias in recall that favoured medical information, treatment and history. This bias within the ward environment has clear advantages for doctors as the focus is on medical, diagnostic and treatment related information. However, it also raises difficulties, as it shows that those aspects of care less easily available to doctors (for the reasons already discussed), for which the doctor is more reliant on their nursing colleagues, appear to be undervalued by those colleagues, not recalled and therefore possibly not reported back to the doctors. The rules that govern which information is valued and passed on within and between nursing and medicine are clearly complex and need much further investigation (Leigh 1987). It does seem, however, that encouragement through actively seeking social and psychological information and valuing all types and aspects of information from colleagues may help ameliorate these problems in communication.

Multidisciplinary team meetings provide a forum for different professionals to voice their opinion about a patient's care. Within many disciplines such as palliative care these meetings work as a forum in which all of those involved in a case can put their perspective, be it physical, social or psychological, and discuss how one aspect may inter-relate to another. This type of forum actively encourages individual professionals to voice opinions and provides a forum for concerns about management to be aired.

Supporting colleagues

A final aspect of communication within health care relates to support of colleagues within and across disciplines. Caring for patients and their families is an emotionally wearing task. Much research has now been published reporting stress, burnout and psychiatric illness in medicine and other health-care disciplines (Ramirez *et al.* 1996; Delvaux *et al.* 1988). Support is therefore a key variable that needs addressing in the workplace.

Interprofessional communication is the key to developing a supportive working environment. We have already discussed the importance of using colleagues to enhance our understanding of patients and to help resolve difficult issues. The role of talking to colleagues, medical and non-medical, about difficult cases in order to gain support is less well acknowledged but equally as important.

There are many aspects of a junior doctor's role that are highly stressful, for example breaking bad news about serious illness, telling someone about a death, or explaining an accident. The stress engendered by these tasks can be shared in the team, medical or multiprofessional, especially if the doctor is not alone when taking on such a task. Thus, joint consultations are not only beneficial for the patients but also provide an ally for the doctor when a conversation is difficult, and can provide a person to share the emotional load with when the conversation has caused distress and tears.

On occasions when a case or its management has been particularly stressful, team debriefings can be of immense benefit. The simple process of sharing how one was feeling, and understanding that others have had similar experiences is not only supportive but also builds relationships within the team, so creating a collective team spirit.

Conclusions

This chapter explores some aspects of how doctors can work effectively with their colleagues with the aim of enhancing patient care. Talking to patients and their relatives is one of the most critical aspects of patient care, and can be one of the most stressful. If that task can be shared, by using the expertise and perspective of our colleagues, then the difficulties of communicating with patients can be made more manageable, and the care we offer our patients enhanced.

References

Anderson, H., Ward, C., Eardley, A., Gomm, S., Connolly, M., Coppinger, T., Corgie, D., Williams, J., Makin, W. (2001). The concerns of patients under palliative care and a heart failure clinic are not being met. *Palliative Medicine*, **15**, 279–86.

Booth, K., Maguire, P., Butterworth, T., Hillier, V.F. (1996). Perceived professional support and the use of blocking behaviours by hospice nurses. *Journal of Advanced Nursing*, **24**, 522–7.

Bornstein, B., Emler, C. (2001). Rationality in medical decisions making: a review of the literature on doctors decision-making biases. *Journal of Evaluation of Clinical Practice*, **7**(2), 97–107.

Bredin, M., Corner, J., Krishnasamy, M., Plant, H., Bailey, C., A'Hearn, R. (1999). Multicentre randomised controlled trial of nursing intervention for breathlessness in patients with lung cancer. *British Medical Journal*, **318**, 901–4.

Cole-Kelly, K. (1992). Illness stories and patients care in the family practice context. *Family Medicine*, **24**, 45–8.

Crow, R., Chase, J., Lamond, D. (1995). The cognitive component of nursing assessment: an analysis. *Journal of Advanced Nursing*, **22**(2), 206–12.

Delvaux, N., Razavi, D., Farvaques, C. (1988). Cancer care—a stress for health professionals. *Social Science and Medicine*, **27**(2), 159–66.

Dowding, D. (2001). Examining the effects that manipulating information given in the change of shift report has on nurses' care planning ability. *Journal of Advanced Nursing*, **33**(6), 836–46.

Dowsett, S.M., Saul, J.L., Butow, P.N., Dunn, S.M., Boyer, M.J., Findlow, R., Dunsmore, J. (2000). Communication style in the cancer consultation: preferences for a patient-centred approach. *Psycho-oncology*, **9**, 147–56.

Fallowfield, L., Lipkin, M., Hall, A. (1998). Teaching senior oncologists communication skills: results from phase 1 of a comprehensive longitudinal program in the United Kingdom. *Journal of Clinical Oncology,* **16**(5), 1961–8.

Fallowfield, L., Jenkins, V., Fareell, V., Saul, J., Duffy, A., Eves, R. (2002). Efficacy of a Cancer Research UK communication skills training model for oncologists: a randomised controlled trial. *Lancet,* **359**, 650–6.

Glajchen, M., Blum, D., Calder, K. (1995). Cancer pain management and the role of social work: barriers and interventions. *Health Social Work,* **20**(3), 200–6.

Girghis, A., Sanson-Fisher, R. (1995). Breaking bad news: consensus guidelines for medical practitioners. *Journal of Clinical Oncology,* **13**, 2449–56.

Hammond, P., Mosley, M. (2002). *Trust Me, I'm a Doctor.* London: Metro Publishing.

Heaven, C.M. (2001). *The Role of Clinical Supervision in Communication Skills Training.* Unpublished PhD thesis, University of Manchester.

Heaven, C.M., Maguire, P. (1997). Disclosure of concerns by hospice patients and their identification by nurses. *Palliative Medicine,* **11**, 283–90.

Heaven, C.M., Maguire, P. (1998). The relationship between patients' concerns and psychological distress in hospice setting. *Psycho-Oncology,* **7**, 502–7.

Higginson, I.J., McCarthy, M. (1993). Validity of the support team assessment schedule: do staff's ratings reflect those made by patients or their families? *Palliative Medicine,* **7**, 219–28.

Jenkins, V.A., Fallowfield, L.J., Poole, K. (2001). Are members of multidisciplinary teams in breast cancer aware of each other's information roles. *Quality in Health Care,* **10**(2), 70–5.

Korsch, B.M., Negrete, V.F. (1972). Doctor–patient communication. *Scientific American,* August, 66–73.

Leigh, H. (1987). Multidisciplinary teams in consultation–liaison psychiatry: the Yale model. *Psychotherapy and Psychosomatics,* **48**(1–4), 83–9.

Ley, P. (1982). Satisfaction, compliance and communication. *British Journal of Clinical Psychology,* **21**, 241–54.

Macleod, R.M. (1991). *Patients with Advanced Breast Cancer: the Nature and Disclosure of Their Concerns.* Unpublished MSc thesis, University of Manchester.

Macleod-Clark, J. (1983). Nurse–patient communication—an analysis of conversations from surgical wards in Nursing research. In *Ten Studies in Patient Care* (Wilson–Barnett, J., ed.). Chichester; John Wiley and Sons.

Madge, S., Khair, K. (2000). Multidisciplinary teams in the United Kingdom: problems and solutions. *Journal of Pediatric Nursing,* **15**(20), 131–4.

Mager, W., Andryowski, M. (2002). Communication in the cancer 'bad news' consultation: patient perceptions and psychological adjustment. *Psycho-oncology,* **11**, 11–46.

Maguire, P. (1985). Improving the detection of psychiatric problems in cancer patients. *Social Science and Medicine,* **20**(8), 819–23.

Maguire, P. (1999). Improving communication with cancer patients. *European Journal of Cancer,* **35**(10), 1415–22.

Maguire, P., Faulkner, A. (1988). Improving the counselling skills of doctors and nurses in cancer care. *British Medical Journal,* **297**, 847–9.

Menzies, I. (1961). *The Functioning of Social Systems as a Defence Against Anxiety: a report on a study of the nursing service of a general hospital,* pp. 3–29. London: Tavistock.

Oberle, K., Hughes, D. (2001). Doctors' and nurses' perceptions of ethical problems in end-of-life decisions. *Journal of Advanced Nursing,* **33**(6), 707–15.

Parker, R., Hopwood, P. (2000). *Literature Review—Quality of life (QL) in black and ethnic minority groups (BEMGs) with cancer.* Report commissioned by Cancer Research UK.

Pennebaker, J.W. (1993). Putting stress into words: health, linguistic and therapeutic implications. *Behavioural Research Therapy,* **31**(6), 539–8.

Pistrang, N., Barker, C. (1992). Disclosure of concerns in breast cancer. *Psycho-oncology,* **1**, 183–92.

Ramirez, A.J., Graham, J., Richards, M.A., Cull, A., Gregory, W.M. (1996). Mental health of hospital consultants: the effects of stress and satisfaction at work. *Lancet,* **347**, 724–8.

Thompson, R. (1995). Participative decision making: Multidisciplinary team involvement in unit design. *AXON,* **17**(2), 46–8.

Wilkinson, S. (1991). Factors which influence how nurses communicate with cancer patients. *Journal of Advanced Nursing,* **16**, 677–88.

Chapter 12

Communication in a multicultural society

Elisabeth Macdonald

Summary

Many different ethnic groups now form important minorities in our community. Sensitivity to matters of cultural importance can greatly enhance doctor–patient relations. Some background of relevance to health issues is given in relation to patients from Muslim, Asian, Jewish, Jehovah's Witness and Afro-Caribbean communities.

General issues

Most Western countries are now home to a wide variety of different peoples, each with their own ethnic identity, culture and religion. Within these minority communities themselves, there may also be wide variation. Followers of any one religion, for example, may differ widely in traditions that developed in their country of origin. Other minority ethnic groups may originate from the same geographical area but differ fundamentally in religious beliefs. Even within groups that are perceived by outsiders as being strongly unified (such as Muslims or Hindus) there may be wide variation, and peoples of similar geographical background may in fact have more in common than religious groupings. Doctors coming into contact with members of minority groups will need to be aware that there exist numerous potential barriers to good communication.

Many members of minority ethnic groups, especially those who grew up abroad in developing countries, will not have had an opportunity for education. For example, studies in Leeds showed that half the Bangladeshi population could neither read nor write English and that 35% could not read or write their own language, Bengali, either (Tufnell *et al.* 1994). When the general level of education is low it is not surprising that knowledge of anatomy, normal physiology or of a specific disease is very scanty indeed. Low levels of education are not only reflected in ignorance of health issues but also in an inability to understand or speak English. Members of the older generation in particular who have come to Britain later in life may have remained isolated within their own community with little opportunity to learn about their new country and its language.

People originating from the Middle East, the Far East and from the Mediterranean have a very strong sense of duty and commitment to family life. Many extended families are almost socially self-sufficient and while this creates a strong sense of security and mutual support, the opportunities for learning are reduced. Parents and children usually keep very close contact throughout life regardless of any differences. When a family member becomes ill then financial and emotional support is unquestioned. Everyone to the best of their ability will want to help. Relatives and friends may for example, want to stay with a patient at all times. Although laudable in many ways, this family presence can be a potential barrier to what British doctors feel is good doctor–patient communication. It is, however, useful to appreciate the extent of the support systems of different cultures and these can greatly facilitate for example a patient's discharge back into the community. Whereas an elderly British patient, normally living alone, may need extensive community support a senior citizen from a different ethnic group may well be welcomed back into the bosom of the family without need of such services as Meals on Wheels on which a British pensioner may depend.

Because of the difficulties posed by lack of opportunity for education and language it is essential that doctors speak in simple non-technical language. It is first worth assessing not only how much English a patient speaks but also how much they understand. It is very much easier to understand a language than to find the vocabulary to speak it oneself. Sentences should be short, clear and precise. In some parts of the world doctors as we know them do not exist. It may therefore be worth explaining your role as a doctor with the strictly professional task of identifying with the patient their health-care needs and agreeing together a programme for clarifying and addressing these problems. It can be helpful for female health-care workers to explain to female patients that male colleagues fulfil this strictly professional role and see the patient as a patient and not as a woman in the usual social sense. Understanding the neutral gender role of a professional can diminish the natural reticence seen in other circumstances that can act as an obstacle to trust.

British people in general, and this applies to health-care professionals also, are sensitive to the expected 'please' and 'thank you' normally attached to a request, but in some countries this may not be the practice. It is worth knowing that there are some languages in which these words do not exist and the omission of these terms of politeness may not therefore represent a deliberate discourtesy.

In recent years the Department of Health has highlighted the ethnic inequalities of health-care provision in Britain (Balarajan and Raleigh 1993). This paper suggests that in order to provide racial equality in health care, professionals need to be more sensitive to the life-styles and cultures of ethnic minority groups as well as being aware of the higher rates of certain diseases within these groups. The quality of care for ethnic minority patients varies greatly across the country due both to access to health services as well as doctor–patient communication.

The bias believed to be at the root of these disparities is nearly always unconscious and typically occurs in hurried situations (Nelson 2003).

Health-care professionals, particularly primary care teams need to be vigilant in early detection and subsequent management of those diseases with high incidence among the local ethnic minority. People from some ethnic minorities, for example, have higher than national rates of diabetes, hypertension, coronary heart disease and stroke with ensuing increased rates of morbidity and mortality. Identifying and controlling hypertension in these groups is the single most effective way of reducing risks (Memon and Abbas 1999). The part played by good communication is clearly fundamental to any initiative for prevention.

Effective detection and improved management of asymptomatic disease such as hypertension will help reduce the recognized poor outcomes of untreated disease. Not only will this vigilance benefit the patient but also at the same time the Health Service itself will benefit financially by reducing the cost of dealing later with the full-blown complications of such disease.

The government public health blueprint *Healthier Nation* (DOH 1998) acknowledges that the chances of living a long and healthy life depend on financial status, location and ethnic background. Britain's South Asian and Afro-Caribbean citizens in particular tend on average to be more socially disadvantaged than the general population. Compared with their indigenous counterparts, the majority of people from ethnic minorities tend more often to live in and around inner cities, tend to have lower socio-economic status and to have greater difficulties of access to health-care services owing to language and cultural barriers. Ensuring equity of health-care access is a challenge for health-care providers everywhere.

A key issue in future health provision remains the approach to health inequalities. Black and South Asian groups often also experience higher morbidity from chronic illness than white groups. One study recently published in the *British Medical Journal*, for example, found that South Asians admitted to hospital with asthma were unclear about many important and fundamental aspects of their condition. They were not aware of how to control the condition, were frequently unfamiliar with the use and benefits of preventative medication and had little confidence in their general practitioner. Those patients reporting difficulty accessing primary care during attacks were more likely to be South Asian in origin. Cultural barriers between patients and clinicians can thus affect the quality of care for chronic illness as well as rates of hospitalization (Griffiths *et al.* 2001).

Health-care professionals need to be aware of prescriptive religious practices and how religious and cultural differences if not handled sensitively can hinder communication. If this subject is approached tactfully and politely it will be welcomed. The importance of respect for each individual cannot be overemphasized. People should be seen as persons in their own right and not simply as culturally typecast. It is already difficult enough for those who are healthy to adjust and fit into a new and alien environment. It is much more difficult for individuals coming from other countries who fall ill and require help and treatment. It is easily forgotten that the medical environment is a doubly alien one in which the patient and their family can be both fearful and confused.

Be aware also that patients from abroad often equate illness with death and doctors need to be aware of this underlying anxiety. In particular, patients from countries where access to health care is restricted may regard as fatal many illnesses that are readily treated in the Western world.

In the compilation of guidance on ethnic diversity a number of issues emerged as being of particular importance or sensitivity. The following list of questions was addressed by a wide variety of colleagues and with sincere thanks and with permission I have listed their names at the end of this chapter. All agreed on the basic premise: greater communication is needed between health-care workers and all patients and their relatives irrespective of ethnic background.

Sensitive cultural questions: topics explored

1. Relationship with doctors. How do members of different cultural groups view doctors and especially doctors of either sex? For example, some women from groups with a different cultural background will have difficulty consulting with and confiding in a male doctor.

2. Death. How is death viewed by different cultural groups? What rituals are associated? What are the family implications arising from the death of a family member?

3. Family structure. Power balance within families and how this may influence doctor–patient relations.

4. Sharing of information. How is information generally communicated within the family, freely or in a strictly hierarchical fashion? Is this related to gender or age?

5. Communication within the cultural group. What are the norms of interpersonal exchange especially as between members of the opposite sex? For example, some communities discourage female members from smiling, making eye contact or removing their veil.

6. Stigma of disease. Attitudes to major diseases such as cancer, tuberculosis and HIV. Are these regarded as shameful diagnoses that result in a patient being shunned and isolated?

7. Misconceptions about health issues. For example, some communities believe that cancer is catching.

8. Marital relationships. Does the husbands' view of his wife's illness have implications for family relationships, sexual relations and fertility, which may create a barrier in doctor–patient relations? Does information communicated by the doctor have potentially damaging implications for the marriage?

9. Age. How does advancing age, with the greater likelihood of poor health, limited medical knowledge, sensitivity and embarrassment affect doctor–patient communication?

10. Community relations. How does each ethnic minority view its place within the wider health community? How open are the ethnic elders to communicate in an open and informative way with the wider society in particular about health-related issues.

Muslim and Arabic speaking families

Islam is the religion of Muslim peoples. It means literally 'submission' signifying that a Muslim is someone who submits to God's will. All Muslims accept the teaching of the holy book the Koran or Quran. Islam, however, is more than a religion. Islam itself is a way of life. It controls politics, local laws, behaviour and every aspect of daily life. It gives guidance in all spheres of human activity from birth to death. Arabic-speaking people are mainly Muslims. There are common features among the 23 Arabic countries though differences exist between regions and result in differing practice and traditions. In addition, there are large Muslim populations in other countries such as Pakistan and Indonesia.

Cultural background

The religious duties incumbent on a practising Muslim are the five 'pillars' of Islam. In summary these are as follows:

1. There is only one God (Allah) and Mohammed is his messenger.
2. Daily prayers are performed five times each day. The Quran commands washing some parts of the body before prayer.
3. A fast from dawn to dusk is observed during the holy month of Ramadan.
4. A donation of charity amounting to 2.5% of every Muslim's wealth is expected and should be given to the needy every year.
5. A pilgrimage, which is called Hajj, to the city of Mecca in Saudi Arabia, is expected once during the lifetime of a Muslim.

Health issues that arise from the practice of Islam

During Ramadan healthy Muslims over the age of 12 fast for approximately 30 days. When fasting no food or drink can be consumed between dawn and sunset and so arrangements need to be made so that food is available during the night. Some very devout Muslims may wish to fast even if they are suffering from poor health. However, the Quran clearly indicates that if a Muslim is very ill the fasting may take place at a more appropriate time. If patients insist on fasting they may request to alter their usual dose or pattern of medicines taking them before beginning the fast each day rather than evenly spacing them throughout the day. It may be possible to address this problem by prescribing slow release medication for some conditions.

The left hand is considered unclean because it is used for bodily ablutions. The right hand is used for eating even if the person is left handed. This should be taken into account when siting intravenous lines and should be discussed with the patient.

In the treatment of diabetes, which is a common condition among Arab peoples, pork insulins, pork-based synthetic insulins and beef (non-halal) insulins are unacceptable to devout Muslims, and human or in fact human-like insulins should be prescribed.

Medical advice is sometimes ignored by devout Muslims for religious reasons and a devoted patient may say for example, 'Allah will protect me.'

He or she may not fear death and may even welcome it in order to meet the Creator sooner. The prophet's teaching, however, encouraged Muslims to see the doctor and comply with treatment and it may be helpful to recruit the help of a religious leader to explain this (Qureshi 2002).

Serious illness and death

Death is perceived and managed differently in the Muslim culture. It is important to take this into consideration when dealing with the sensitive issues of death and bereavement. Like Christians and Jews, Muslims believe in life after death merely as one stage in God's overall plan for humanity. Devout and pious Muslims believe that death is to be seen as a temporary separation from the family and that this is God's will. It is for this reason that some Muslims discipline themselves to show no emotion at a death because it would suggest rebellion against God's will. It is, however, much more common to find grief being openly displayed.

In Islam illness is regarded as a test of how strongly a person believes in God. If he endures the illness with fortitude this proves him to be a true believer. Even when a person is very ill it is still believed that God has the power to revive him. This leads to the view that no treatment should ever be discontinued and this can cause conflict between medical carers and patients and families.

In Islam it is not acceptable to discontinue any treatment that has any chance of success in reviving the patient no matter how remote. Some families do not like to be warned of impending death. They feel that because you are telling them about death you may be likely to interfere and contribute to that death.

It is believed that if the patient is to die it is the will of God and the doctor should not think that he knows God's mind. The doctor should not believe that he knows what God intends. It is an Islamic belief that both the day you are born and the day you will die have been foretold. The belief is that when that day comes the individual will die and there is nothing that can be done to prevent this because it is God's will.

Longer life is viewed as valuable under Islam. It is believed that the longer a person lives the greater is the time to carry out good deeds in God's name. The benefit of long life lies in the opportunity to do a greater number of acts of wisdom and generosity, which will improve a person's outlook in the after life. Death itself is accepted as a means to a greater purpose.

It is another tenet of Islam that each family member must do his best for a relative and this means the maximum effort that each can sustain. A truly devout Muslim believes that he must not give up on anything ever. Eventually the will of God will prevail. This affects everything in life and not just the practice of medicine and terminal care.

How can this Muslim view of terminal care, that every possible available treatment and resuscitation procedure must be attempted, be reconciled with the guidelines for intensive care and cardiopulmonary resuscitation outlined in Chapter 6? In discussions concerning the appropriateness of cardiopulmonary resuscitation the family will naturally expect that a full attempt at resuscitation will be carried out. The family will not want to accept the responsibility of allowing a decision not to resuscitate. Their duty is the protection of the patient and pursuit of any chance of life no matter how small. Many Muslim families may feel that the availability of life support, which is not possible in their country of origin, demands that their relative should be given every possible benefit.

Senior doctors of the Muslim faith in Britain recommend that it is wise to continue those procedures of support or treatment that are not harmful to the patient. Simple measures such as intravenous fluids should be carried on for the patient's welfare because it is comforting to the family to know that simple supportive measures are continuing. These simple measures apart the same guidelines apply.

Gender

Islam teaches that women and men are regarded almost as equal. They have the same duties, prayers and fasting. Exceptions are made for women who are pregnant or during their period. Men do tend to dominate their women but this is not actually a written injunction of the Quran. Male dominance comes more from custom and varies between communities. Arabic men do tend to dominate women to some degree but less stringently than, for example, the male population of Pakistan. Male clerics proclaim that this is part of the Quran but in reality it is custom rather than teaching. The text of the Quran is liable to interpretation in many contexts and teachers who interpret the Quran gain followers whose views coincide.

It is customary for members of the opposite sex to avoid eye contact for reasons of modesty. In accordance with the commands of the Quran many Muslim women cover their heads with a veil or cover their entire bodies. To some extent Muslim men and women are kept segregated. Particularly in the X-ray department Muslims may be offended if asked to change into a gown and sit in a public area prior to examination. Sometimes a male patient will request only a male nurse or radiographer, not because they do not like females but they do not wish to cause offence. In Arabic cultures most patients prefer a doctor of the same sex and this is especially true for women.

Privacy is considered very important and permission must be sought before entering a room. Muslim families will expect the doctor or nurse to knock before entering and wait for a response before going in. A pause between knocking and entering gives female family members time to cover themselves if they wish. The habit in Britain of doctors knocking and entering immediately can cause considerable offence. Nakedness and unfamiliar Western clothes can be a source of considerable distress especially among the elderly, and care must be taken within reason to show respect in the way we ourselves are dressed. Short skirts, naked arms and low necklines will not be thought compatible with professional conduct in most cultures including our own!

Sharing information

Many Arabic and Muslim families do not like the patient to know when a serious diagnosis has been made. Cancer, for example, is regarded as a death sentence and is very frightening in Arabic countries. Families fear that the patient will refuse treatment and give up altogether if they know the diagnosis. In similar circumstances it should be said many British families may also prefer to have the truth softened a little.

When dealing with a serious diagnosis such as cancer many Muslim families will seek to obscure the truth. Alternative terms are used such as that of a 'serious infection' for which 'strong treatment' is needed. The word cancer itself is usually avoided. However, the younger generation are more open and more likely to ask direct questions. When any other diagnosis is appropriate and the condition is not life threatening then the more explanation that is volunteered the better.

Some Arabic families prefer to consult a non-Arabic speaking doctor because the family can then be sure that the doctor will not discuss the true diagnosis with the patient. This leaves the management of information concerning diagnosis and treatment in the hands of the family and this can be problematic for doctors who feel that the ethical principle of patient autonomy should be sacrosanct. Careful and sensitive negotiation is required to reconcile the family's demand for secrecy with the patient's right to an appropriate level of self-determination. It can be argued, however, that the patient will feel safest within the cultural guidelines with which he is familiar and will come to his or her own solution in the knowledge that his family is likely to be protecting him from any news they think he will find unwelcome. If the patient chooses to press the doctor and to seek more definitive information then the opportunity will arise for a fuller level of disclosure.

One charming story illustrates the way in which Muslims believe God encourages initiative and perseverance.

> One day, seeking guidance, a Bedouin came to visit Mohammed in his tent. Without delay he dismounted from his camel and hastened into the tent. When Mohammed asked the Bedouin if he had tethered his precious camel, the Bedouin replied that 'No, he had not. He had left the camel in the safe hands of God.'
>
> Mohammed reportedly replied, 'You should first tie up your camel and then leave it to Allah!'

In other words for a Muslim it is necessary to behave with care and wisdom that God will then reward!

Patients from the Indian subcontinent

Cultural background

Recently arrived immigrant families from India, Pakistan and Bangladesh now form sizeable minority groups in many cities in the UK. In India there are several regional languages but Hindi is commonly understood. In Pakistan the commonly spoken language is Urdu. Spoken Urdu and Hindi are very similar but they differ in their script. Urdu script is similar to Arabic and Persian and written from right to left, whereas Hindi and Bengali scripts are written from the left to right. Bangladeshis speak the Bengali language but some can also understand Urdu and Hindi. The majority of Pakistanis and Bangladeshis are Muslim while Hindus are the majority in India. Culturally, there are striking similarities among the people of the Indian subcontinent and many of the people coming from this region are well versed in English and Western tradition. However, education may have been rudimentary and older patients from these communities may neither speak English nor understand the role of a doctor.

Currently, the leaders and elders of Asian minorities report that feedback from their community describes doctor–patient communication in many areas as almost non-existent. The challenge for us all is to rectify this regrettable deficiency.

Health issues that arise among Asian minority groups

Bengali families tend to be fatalistic. The head of the family is usually the eldest male and this, for example, may be an uncle rather than the father of the patient concerned. Female elders are also respected in Hindu and Bengali cultures. The Asian family, however, is hierarchical. Information is strictly controlled and Asian patients tend not to tell their extended families nor their community about health issues. Being fatalistic these patients fear that they will die and would rather not be surrounded by the doom and gloom, which tends to engulf families of the sick.

Health information is often strictly controlled within the close family. What is considered the 'nuclear' family among Asian communities, however, differs from the European view. In Asian families roles in a sense overlap. Brothers, sisters and cousins are brought up together often in the same household. An aunt fulfils a similar role to the mother. There is thus little distinction between siblings and cousins.

Different assumptions are therefore normal concerning confidentiality and involvement. Whereas in Britain a doctor would expect to talk to the patient and his or her spouse only, among Asian families a family conference may be called. From a practical point of view this can only be useful. When serious matters need discussion the family will decide who comes and how responsibility will be shared. Family duty is considered very important and extends across generations. It is, for example, the son's duty to care for his mother and this may include paying for private medical care even when the son still remains in the Indian subcontinent.

When planning a patient's future care it is essential to take into consideration the potential of extended family support both in the hospital and at home. Where financial deprivation does not prevent it the care plan should involve the family at each stage. Active family support will enable a patient to return home from a hospital stay earlier and the usual provisions for 'risk assessment' before discharge may be quite inappropriate. Unnecessarily long inpatient care can be safely avoided to the benefit of the patient and the NHS.

Gender

Husbands tend to talk to each other about matters of importance rather than to their wives. Women in immigrant Asian families on the other hand often tend to be very isolated. They are discouraged from travelling alone on public transport and as their husband often uses the car for work there is no easy way for them to attend hospital, health education or language classes.

Fertility is highly valued among Asian families and the prospect of hysterectomy, especially among young women, is a delicate matter. Men tend to regard infertile women as being of little value even although they may already have proven their fertility and produced several children.

Serious illness and death

Some illnesses such as cancer carry with them a stigma but more as a result of ignorance than as a matter of shame. Asian radio and television is doing much to educate immigrant families and young Asians tend to be very hard working and motivated. Families of sick patients prefer to isolate themselves from the community. This is a self-imposed isolation rather than a matter of being shunned by the community. Attitudes among the less-educated Asians are similar to those pertaining in Victorian days in the UK. The sick tend to be kept out of sight and a young wife who becomes ill may in fact be sent back to her own family. Asian families are, however, emerging slowly into the community and are beginning to avail themselves of health services. The elderly on the other hand may know so little that they don't know what they don't know. In contrast, some attitudes are refreshingly positive. Some families prefer to be fiercely independent and assert that it is not the responsibility of the NHS to reach out to them but rather their responsibility to inform themselves. They feel they should learn to get help just like anyone else (Dr Kulsum Winship 2002, personal communication).

Cancer remains a fearful diagnosis among Asian families. Some husbands knowing that cancer is relatively rare among women in the subcontinent reject the possibility that their own wife could develop the disease. The incidence of breast cancer in the Indian subcontinent is indeed two to three times lower than in Britain but life expectancy is also lower. Asian women of breast screening age are mainly first generation immigrants and would be expected to have a lower incidence than the indigenous population. This observation is borne out by studies in the UK (Matheson et al. 1984; Barker and Baker 1990). However, the incidence of cancer in minority groups is expected to rise as a result of increased exposure to risk factors especially in the second and subsequent generations adopting Western life-styles (Raleigh and Payne 1993). In the USA for instance the risk among Asian settlers has doubled within a decade.

One result of cultural difference is that many immigrant communities would rather use Ayurvedic or other alternative medicines before seeking conventional medical advice. This choice can act as a potent barrier to early access to medical care and cause delay in Asian families seeking appropriate orthodox medical care for serious conditions (LSHTM 2001). A recent study in East London, for example, revealed that many Bengali women are still presenting with very advanced stages of breast cancer. Although in the UK breast cancer survival rates have improved, there is still a large difference in deaths within 6 months of diagnosis between the UK and other European countries. This cannot be explained by treatment differences alone and is likely to reflect delayed presentation, for example, among Asian women (Purushotham et al. 2001).

A further complication arising from the use of Ayuverdic therapies may occur when these therapies continue to be used in addition to conventional Western medicine with the risk of unidentified interactions.

Death

Perhaps what Hindus would value most of all from their doctors is an appreciation of the cultural sensitivity and rituals relating to death and burial. Unlike the practice of the Jewish and Muslim religions there is not, among Hindus, the urgency of burying their dead before nightfall. Most Hindus are in fact cremated in accordance with ancient custom. It is traditional to cremate as soon as possible. However, in the UK the cremation ceremony may be delayed by a few days to ensure that it can take place at a crematorium that is closer to home or more accessible or while waiting for close relatives living abroad to reach the UK. This of course can delay the psychological recovery process as the cremation is another painful experience in addition to the death itself that the relatives must endure.

Considerable distress can be caused by inattention to devout observance of death and mourning. While understandably preoccupied with working for the living a junior doctor who postpones completing a death certificate may be oblivious of the anguish caused to a religious family by such delay.

Some religious groups for whom bodily integrity is important find the request for a post-mortem examination anathema and totally unacceptable. Sensitive negotiation will be needed when this examination is at the coroner's behest.

Since the Alderhay Enquiry into the retention of body parts the public has been made rudely aware of the necessity for post-mortem examination and retention of organs for legal or scientific reasons (Independent Review Group on Retention of Organs at Post Mortem). The continuation of many valuable lines of research may depend on regaining the confidence of the public in the probity of this procedure. Much misunderstanding and conflict could be averted by more open discussion of the possible need to broach this issue with a family in the event of death.

The language barrier remains the most important impediment to health access for immigrant Asian families. It is essential for doctors and nurses to speak slowly, clearly and in simple terms avoiding technical vocabulary. Signs and leaflets in the patient's own native language are invaluable in explaining such alien concepts as the doctors role, what to expect at a hospital visit, what is involved in different investigations and how to obtain further information. Many big city hospitals are now well geared to providing this multilingual support. In view of the high degree of illiteracy among Asian immigrants for whom written information is unhelpful some hospitals, for example in Bradford, have produced audiotapes of information and videotapes in different languages (Tufnell *et al.* 1994). In addition, some Hindu Temples and other centres of worship have taken a valuable lead in promoting health issues among their own congregation. Health-care panels have been appointed from trained members of the community. The primary objectives are twofold: first, to educate their society in the use of mainstream services, and secondly to screen for those serious diseases such as heart disease, which are prevalent in that society. Some temples have welcomed mobile breast screening units staffed by a female team. Thus some Asian women can have confidence that they will be treated under temple protection with cultural sensitivity. What is important is the need to tailor the service to local needs (N. Shah 2003, personal communication).

Asians vary in their degree of integration and thus in their health-care requirements. Intermarriage with other communities is increasing and with this trend the sense of isolation will diminish with time. The younger generation are becoming more informed about health issues and access. They have also developed more confidence in persuading their elders to seek help. There is, however, a long way to go to reach equal access and treatment and health-care professionals must remain vigilant, without being patronizing, that health messages are understood.

One further problem is often unrecognized when dealing with second-generation immigrant patients and relatives. This group has been born and brought up in the UK and have often adopted values similar to those of the host community. However, they are also brought up in a traditional home environment where the values and expectations may be very different. Stressful situations such as illness and death exacerbate this clash of values and beliefs. Doctors need to be alert to such problems and help the different generations to air their views and reconcile the differences by negotiation.

Jewish patients and their families

In Britain today there is a diversity of opinion ranging from Liberal through Reform, Orthodox and ultra Orthodox Jewish faith. Liberal, Reform and Orthodox Jewish opinion in medical matters tends to reflect that of the wider community. However, ultra Orthodox Jews tend to live in a much more closed community and manifest more traditional views. Approximately 300 000 Jewish people currently live in Britain.

Relations with doctors

Most Jewish patients are happy to see a doctor of either sex. However, this may not apply to Orthodox Jewish patients who would prefer to see a doctor of the same sex. In previous years the traditional Jewish family was closely knit and part of a matriarchy supervised by a powerful older Jewish woman. Jewish women in the past have tended to outlive their husbands. However, the days of extended Jewish families have largely gone. Most Jewish people are fairly well integrated into the rest of the community and, although this is less claustrophobic, it does mean that there is less support available to the individual. Previously, a wise member of the family would be available to 'listen' and 'counsel' relatives with problems, but young people in particular are now more isolated.

Within the Jewish community doctors are still respected. The older generation will respect the doctor for his learning while the younger generation will judge on performance. The older generation tend to be afraid of doctors and delay going to see the doctor because they don't want to bother him. They have both a respect for and a fear of medicine and are frightened by doctors. This probably stems from a fear of what the doctor may tell them in terms of 'The Disease', 'The Big C', or in other words cancer. It is usually the younger members of the family who persuade their relative to consult a doctor. The young, however, can be anxious and fearful about health issues and seek support from their family practitioner in place of a sympathetic relative as in days gone by.

Death

It is normal for a member of the Orthodox Jewish community to be buried within 1 or 2 days. This is normally within an Orthodox Jewish burial ground. Those from the Liberal and Reformed synagogues, however, accept cremation. Following death a body should not be touched by non-Jewish people and a family member will attend to sit with the body. The body is often washed and prepared for burial by special Jewish attendants. In the Jewish faith it is important that the body is buried intact and for this reason post-mortem examination is not encouraged. It is important to be sensitive when discussing the necessity for post-mortem examination after a sudden death. The idea of post-mortem investigation can cause considerable distress to an orthodox family and it is important in these circumstances to negotiate sensitively with a family representative. Following the night of burial relatives will 'sit shiva' for 7 days. This is a gathering of family and friends each evening when special prayers are spoken (Kaddish). Mourners sit on low chairs without a cushion and candles are lit each evening. Candles are also lit on the anniversary of the death each year (Yahrzeit candle). It is normal for orthodox males not to shave until the period of mourning is over.

People react to death in different ways. Towards the end it is sensible to find out quietly from a close family representative what should be done in the event of death and who should be contacted. Flowers are not appropriate at a Jewish funeral.

Family structure

The Jewish family can be a minefield of complex inter-relations. Often every member of the family wants to be involved and to know what is going on. It is wise to meet with the closest relatives and sit in conference with them to explore the feelings both of the patient and the family. Sometimes the true diagnosis may be hidden from family members and it is important to be sensitive to the patient's wishes about the sharing of information. The patient may need to be shielded to some degree from family members who attempt to be obsessively controlling. On the other hand it is wise to be clear with whom you are communicating in the family and refer other family members to this representative. As far as is possible do be forthcoming and communicative within the parameters expressed by the patient.

Gender

It is not uncommon for Orthodox Jewish males to avoid shaking hands with members of the opposite sex. On the whole women are not encouraged to fraternize with men outside the family. At the time of their marriage Orthodox Jewish women shave their head entirely and will keep the head shaved for the rest of their life. The head is, however, covered by a wig known as a Sheitl, which, however, is often very stylish and fashionable. The Jewish faith is not a proselytizing religion. Many Jewish young people now marry 'out' in other words a non-Jewish partner. As with most minority groups the Jewish community is becoming more integrated and absorbed into wider British society.

Husbands may interfere in the doctor–patient relationship and seek to control the medical management of their wives. Women tend to talk quite openly while men are less communicative. It is common for married Jewish couples to avoid intercourse, before, during and immediately after a woman's period and in the orthodox community matters of sexuality, fertility and reproduction are regarded as highly sensitive and private matters.

Old age

Many elderly Jewish patients do not feel comfortable talking to young doctors especially of the opposite sex. There is a custom of privacy that tends to make older patients embarrassed about discussing their own bodies. They will also tend to tell the doctor what they think the doctor wants to hear.

Often Jewish patients will ask to be told the truth but in fact may really be seeking to hear what they would like to hear rather than the truth itself. It is wise to feel your way gently in these circumstances and to tune in carefully to help you estimate how much the patient really wants you to tell them.

One practical difficulty arising from the practice of the Jewish faith, especially for the elderly, is that during the fast day of Yom Kippur, which extends from sunset to sunset and lasts 25 hours, Orthodox and observant Jewish people will refrain not only from taking food and liquid but also from taking their medication. This can lead to severe medical problems, for example cardiac complications, when needed medication is suddenly discontinued.

Orthodox Jewish teaching in fact stipulates that religious observance should not be allowed to harm the individual's health but this is reportedly not well known among the Jewish community (Adrian Whiteson 2003, personal communication).

Elderly people tend to be treated with respect and dignity among the Jewish community and this respect should be extended to the elderly of all groups in our society.

Jehovah's Witnesses

Most health-care professionals know one important fact concerning the beliefs of Jehovah's Witnesses, namely that blood transfusion is against their religious beliefs. The Witnesses are a Christian religious group founded in 1872 in Pittsburgh Pennsylvania by an American clergyman, Charles Taze Russell. The governing body of Jehovah's Witnesses is the Watchtower Bible and Tract society of Pennsylvania. Members of the group believe in the second coming of Christ. They regard themselves as practitioners of primitive Christianity and consider each Witness a minister. Jehovah's Witnesses stress bible study and absolute obedience to biblical precepts. The group's teachings are spread primarily by members who preach from door to door. Witnesses acknowledge allegiance solely to the kingdom of Jesus Christ. They refuse consequently to salute any flag, perform military service, vote or otherwise signify allegiance to any government. This policy has brought them into conflict with governmental authorities in many countries. In the late 1990s the world membership of active adherents was reported by the Jehovah's Witnesses to be 5.9 million.

Witnesses are deeply religious people who believe that blood transfusion is forbidden for them by biblical passages such as: 'Only flesh with its soul—its blood—you must not eat' (Genesis 9: 3–4), or 'You must pour its blood out and cover it with dust' (Leviticus 17: 13–14). While these verses are not stated in medical terms Witnesses view them as ruling out transfusion of whole blood, packed red blood cells and plasma as well as white blood cells and platelet administration. However, Witnesses' religious understanding does not absolutely prohibit the use of components such as albumin, immune globulins and haemophiliac preparations. Each Witness must decide individually if he can accept these (The Watch Tower 1978). Witnesses believe that blood removed from the body should be disposed of, and this means that they do not accept auto-transfusion of pre-donated blood. Some otherwise conscientious Witnesses do, however, reject official Watchtower Society blood policy (Elder 2000).

Doctors therefore face a special challenge in treating Jehovah's Witnesses. However, medical personnel need not be concerned about medical negligence liability as Jehovah's Witnesses are very willing to acknowledge their informed refusal of blood.

Although formerly many doctors and hospital officials viewed refusal of transfusion as a legal problem and sought court authorization to proceed, more recent medical literature reveals that a change in attitude occurred during the 1980s. This may be as a result of more surgical experience with patients having very low haemoglobin levels but may also reflect increased awareness of the legal principle of informed consent (Dixon and Smalley 1981). Now large numbers of elective surgical and trauma cases involving both adults and minors are being managed without blood transfusion. Recently, representatives of Jehovah's Witnesses have initiated dialogue with the medical profession in order to improve understanding and help resolve questions about blood salvage, transplants and the avoidance of medico-legal confrontations. Although surgeons have often declined to treat Witnesses because their stand on the use of blood products seems to 'tie the doctors' hands', many doctors have now chosen to view the situation as only one more complication challenging their skill.

As Witnesses do not object to colloid or crystalloid replacement fluids, nor to electrocautery, hypotensive anaesthesia, or hypothermia these have been employed successfully (Dixon and Smalley 1981). In 1977 Ott and Cooley for example reported on 542 cardiovascular operations performed on Witnesses without transfusing blood and concluded that this procedure can be done 'with an acceptably low risk'.

Care of children presents the greatest concern and in the past often resulted in legal action against parents under child neglect legislation. However, this approach is currently questioned by both doctors and lawyers familiar with Witness cases. In all other ways Witness parents seek good medical care for their children and are not desirous of shirking their parental responsibility or of shifting it to a judge or other third party. Within the bounds of the child's best interests the safe management of the young patient needs to be negotiated while respecting firmly held religious views no matter how misguided these may seem to the health-care team.

It is axiomatic that parents have a voice in the care of their children such as when the risk/benefit potentials of surgery, radiation or chemotherapy are faced. A Witness parent simply asks that therapies be used that are not religiously prohibited. This accords with the medical tenet of treating 'the whole person' and not overlooking the possible psychosocial damage of an invasive procedure that violates the family's fundamental beliefs with lasting consequences.

Rather than consider the Witness patient a problem, more and more doctors, at least in the USA, seem to accept the situation as a medical challenge. In meeting the challenge they have developed a standard of practice for this group of patients. Witnesses recognize that, medically, their firmly held conviction appears to add a degree of risk and may complicate their care. Accordingly, they often manifest unusual appreciation for the care they receive. In addition to having both deep faith and an intense will to live, they gladly cooperate with physicians and medical staff.

It is clear that refusal of treatment adds particular challenges to the delivery of compassionate care (Knuti 2002). While respecting a person's autonomy, it is none the less uncomfortable for most health-care professionals to watch the patients deny themselves what staff regard as simple and potentially life-saving measures. You will probably encounter a Witness family at some stage in your career so it is as well to understand the core beliefs.

The Afro-Caribbean community

Within the Afro-Caribbean community there is a wide variety of geographical backgrounds and countries of origin. Within Africa alone there is enormous variation between the cultures of, for example Kenya, Nigeria and South Africa all of whom none the less have historical British connections. The Caribbean Islands, which were of course partly populated by slaves abducted from West Africa during the nineteenth century, are equally varied. Attitudes to doctors and medical practice therefore vary widely. It is worth noting that the Afro-Caribbean community is not generally hampered by the same language barrier that creates difficulties for other ethnic minority groups.

Attitude to doctors

Among some of the older members of the Afro-Caribbean community there may be mistrust of the medical profession. The older generation may still have some suspicions about the motives of white doctors as a result of past stories of the use of black people for experimentation in early drug trials. The most notorious of these trials was known as The Tuskegee Syphilis Experiment. In 1932 a group of scientists secretly selected 400 black people from Tuskegee, Alabama who were never told that they had syphilis but were observed off treatment even when Penicillin became available to treat the condition. The experiment was stopped only when the American public was alerted to it and President Clinton eventually made a public apology to the eight remaining survivors in May 1997 (Brawley 1998; Corbie-Smith 1999; Konotey-Ahulu 2003).

However, although this suspicion persists in the USA there are now fourth generation Afro-Caribbean citizens in the UK among whom these attitudes are no longer typical. The employment of many black doctors and nurses in the NHS has further helped in changing the perception of the hospital community. One effective way of building confidence is for the health-care team to involve staff belonging to the same ethnic group to explain the team's intentions.

Suspicions between the races, however, do go both ways and just as black patients may have some hesitations about consulting a white doctor, so white patients may hesitate to consult a black physician.

Family and gender

In common with many other cultures women often feel more comfortable consulting a woman doctor. Similarly, men feel more comfortable talking to a male. This can be particularly relevant in certain potentially embarrassing situations. For example, sickle cell anaemia is most commonly seen among patients of African origin. Impaired passage of red cells through the microcirculation leads to obstruction of small vessels and one complication can be that of painful priapism (penile erection). Male patients with this condition are understandably reticent about discussing with female staff their concerns about such a personal sexual problem (I. Okpala, Consultant in Charge, Sickle Cell Unit, St Thomas' Hospital London, 2003, personal communication).

In common with most traditional societies men have been excluded from the delivery room and there have been no male midwives. This has changed recently with the development of gynaecology and obstetrics as medical specialities.

In Africa it is of extreme importance for a woman to bear a baby boy and women who fail to produce a son carry the blame for this failure. This is regarded not only as a personal misfortune but has wider implications for the welfare of the whole family.

Many Afro-Caribbean patients may be poorly informed on sexual matters and it is worth knowing that some Caribbean men have quite aggressive feelings towards homosexuality. This in turn means that personal examination and especially rectal examination may be very difficult for Caribbean men to accept. If rectal examination is essential then it is necessary to explain clearly why this examination is necessary and to seek explicit consent.

Attitudes to death

Death is viewed as a great loss among the Afro-Caribbean community even when the person was of advanced years. Death is rarely regarded as a relief but rather as a tragedy, which is mourned openly. During the acute stages of mourning condolence visitors join with the family to grieve openly with tears, dancing and singing. When these visitors leave the sadness of those bereaved may be all the more profound.

In the event of the death of a family breadwinner the sons and uncles will take over the responsibility and an uncle may, for example, act as a family 'regent'.

Sharing information

Information is freely communicated among senior family members. The young may be spared the trauma of harsh facts until they are old enough to cope with them or in an emergency until there is sufficient family support in place. Following a death, sons are rapidly and preferentially informed in order that funeral arrangements can be made. A son may also be sent as a diplomatic messenger to bring bad news to other family members rather than breaking news abruptly by telephone.

Stigma of disease

Among the Afro-Caribbean community it can be the fear of death that motivates attitudes to disease. It is not regarded as shameful to have a disease but the fear of this illness being communicated and causing death in the community may lead to the sick being avoided, although they are no longer shunned. However, because of the fear of 'catching' any disease it is essential that doctors and the nursing staff are careful how they communicate with friends and relatives. Indiscreet choice of language may inadvertently lead to your patient being isolated and unsupported in their community.

Age

Age is respected in most African and Caribbean communities. The elders of the community have an important role in health education that, however, is not often exercised.

One issue that has recently been highlighted through community elders and the Church is the disinclination of the black community to donate either blood or organs for transplantation. Blood is viewed as, in a sense, the very life of the person and the donation of blood is consequently seen as giving part of your own life. Blood is therefore very emotive and even fairly minor injuries involving blood loss can cause panic. However, as communities become better informed the blood donation rate rises. This is more a question of information rather than tradition.

Members of the Afro-Caribbean community, because of the high incidence of hypertensive heart failure and renal failure among this group, are major recipients of organ donation. Until recently virtually no black donors were found. However, community leaders have voiced a strong call to their adherents to reconsider this position on the basis of 'spiritual reciprocity' saying that a community should not receive if not prepared to give. Similarly, up to now donors of bone marrow rarely volunteer from this community. As a consequence bone marrow transplantation for community members using riskier matched unrelated donors is more common leading in turn to greater need for donation of appropriate blood groups and an overall poorer outcome.

Acknowledgements

My thanks are due in addition to the following contributors to this chapter: Dr M. Mohammed, Dr Ayoub Ayoub-Bey, Prof. F.I.D. Kotoney-Ahulu, Dr I. Okpala, Dr Kulsum Winship, Dr N. Shah, Dr A. Whiteson, Suresh Ramburan RN and Dr David Treacher.

References

Balarajan, R., Raleigh, V.S. (1993). *Ethnicity and Health: a guide for the NHS*. London: Department of Health.

Barker, R.M., Baker, M.R. (1990). Incidence of cancer in Bradford Asians. *Journal of Epidemiology and Community Health*, **44**, 125–9.

Brawley, O.W. Office of Special Populations Research, National Cancer Institute, Bethesda, Maryland. (1998). The study of untreated syphilis in the Negro male. *International Journal of Radiation Oncology, Biology, Physics*, **40**, 5–8.

Corbie-Smith, G. (1999). The continuing legacy of the Tuskegee Syphilis study: considerations for clinical investigation. *American Journal of the Medical Sciences*, **317**, 5–8.

Dixon, J.L., Smalley, M.G. (1981). Jehovah's Witnesses and the surgical/ethical challenge. *Journal of the American Medical Association*, **246**(21), 2471–2.

Elder, L. (2000). Why some Jehovah's Witnesses reject official Watchtower Society blood policy. *Journal of Medical Ethics*, **26**, 375–80.

Griffiths, C., Kaur, G., Gantley, M., Feder, G., Hillier, S., Goddard, J., Packe, G. (2001). Influences on hospital admission for asthma in south Asian and white adults: qualitative interview study. *British Medical Journal*, **323**, 962–26.

Independent Review Group on Retention of Organs at Post Mortem: Final Report http://www.show.scot.nhs.uk/sehd/scotorgrev/Final%20Report/ropm–02.htm

Knuti, K.A., Amrein, P.C., Chabner, B.A., Lynch, T.J. Jnr, Penson, R.T. (2002). Faith, identity, and leukaemia: when blood products are not an option. *Oncologist*, **7**(4), 371–80.

Konotey-Ahulu, F.I.D. (2003). The politics of AIDS in South Africa: beyond the controversies. Rapid response BMJ website. *British Medical Journal*, **326**, 495–7.

LSHTM (London School of Hygiene and Tropical Medicine) Cancer and Public Health Unit and Macmillan Cancer Relief Report. (2001). An Investigation of the Barriers and Enablers to Early Presentation in Disadvantaged Groups.

Matheson, M., Dunnigan, M.G., Hole, D., Gillis, C.R. (1984). Incidence of colo-rectal, breast and lung cancer in a Scottish Asian population. *Health Bulletin*, **43**, 245–9.

Memon, M., Abbas, F. (1999). Reducing health risks in ethnic communities. *Nursing Times*, **95**(27), 48–50.

Nelson, A. (2003). Chair: The Institute of Medicine Report, Unequal treatment: Confronting racial and ethnic disparities in healthcare. Perception vs. Reality. American Medical Association website, www.ama-assn.org

Ott, D.A., Cooley, D.A. (1977). Cardiovascular surgery in Jehovah's witnesses. *Journal of the American Medical Association*, **238**, 1256–8.

Purushotham, A.D., Pain, S.J., Miles, D., Harnett, A. (2001). Variations in treatment and survival in breast cancer. *Lancet Oncology*, **2**(12), 719–25.

Qureshi, B. (2002). Diabetes in Ramadan. *Journal of the Royal Society of Medicine*, **95**, 489–90.

Raleigh, V.S., Payne, A. (1993). Cancer among black and ethnic populations. Health and Race—creating social change. Kings Fund in collaboration with University of Surrey. pp. 1–3. Fact sheet no. 5.

Shah, N. (2003). Personal communication.

Tufnell, D.J., Nuttall, K., Raistrick, J., Jackson, T.L. (1994). Use of translated written material to communicate with non-English speaking patients. British Medical Journal, **309**, 992.

Chapter 13

Apologies in clinical medicine

Carmel O'Donovan

Summary

It is always hard to admit fault and an apology requires courage and insight. When this exchange is in the face of a clinical incident with ongoing sequelae there can be many additional valid concerns with regard to issues such as liability, i.e. 'Who will pay?' if things have gone wrong and a patient has been harmed. This chapter seeks to demystify the area of apology and to offer strategies that will minimize problems for both the health-care provider and the patient. It deals with the fundamentals of legal liability and looks at the ways in which clinical risk management and governance underpin patient protection mechanisms.

It concludes with three real life cases that serve to illustrate the points made in the: What does it mean to say sorry? What constitutes a valid apology and what implications does this have for the doctor, his employer and the patient?

The dictionary defines an apology as a verbal or written expression of regret or contrition for a fault or failing. No one who has watched the film *A Fish Called Wanda* can every forget the apology issued by Archie Leach . . .

Archie: All right, all right, I apologize.

Otto: You're really sorry!

Archie: I'm really really sorry, I apologize unreservedly.

Otto: You take it back!

Archie: I do, I offer a complete and utter retraction. The imputation was totally without basis in fact, and was in no way fair comment, and was motivated purely by malice, and I deeply regret any distress that my comments may have caused you, or your family, and I hereby undertake not to repeat any such slander at any time in the future.

Otto: OK.

The fact that this apology was elicited by Archie being hung by his ankles from a high building may detract somewhat from its value and is not intended to imply that this is the way in which the medical profession should approach the serious issue of what to say when things go wrong.

In the words of the Elton John song 'Don't it seem to go . . . sorry seems to be the hardest word?'

Introduction

In the main, the issue of acknowledging a problem, apologizing and empathizing with the patient can prove difficult to many doctors and health-care providers:

- They may themselves have mixed emotions about the events, which have taken place.
- They may feel vulnerable and threatened.
- They may question their own competence and clinical future.
- They may fear that they will be castigated if an apology is made as a claim may follow.

For all of these reasons doctors may try to hide behind a wall of silence. This leaves them and the patient as long-term casualties of an untoward incident. No one benefits from this attitude and it is an essential part of clinical practice to be aware of this.

In recommending that an apology is offered where there has been an adverse outcome is in the patient and the clinician's best interests, it is important to be mindful that while an apology is not a legal admission of liability, a patient seeking legal advice having been offered an apology may be advised that the legal perspective is that an apology has two parts: First, as an expression of regret, and secondly as a tacit acceptance of responsibility.

Thus in making an apology the clinician need to be mindful of the value of saying enough to express regret without committing his employers to any legal liability unless and until it can be shown that this is an appropriate part of the 'apology package'. This latter aspect of the assessment of the untoward incident is likely to involve an independent overview of the event and may take some time, although every effort should be made to expedite this process.

Of note in this context is the recent development, which will place doctors and managers in the NHS under a statutory 'duty of candour' requiring them to tell patients of negligent acts or omissions causing harm. This new NHS 'redress' scheme is intended to avoid the need for the costly adversarial process usually associated with medical negligence claims. It is also intended to end the 'blame culture' feared by clinical staff reporting negligent acts.

Clinical risk management and governance

It has become a fundamental part of the process of care delivery to be able to demonstrate that a system of clinical risk management exists within the health-care setting.

The clinical risk management process involves the systematic identification assessment and reduction of harm to patients. It is thus incumbent on health-care providers to develop systems for reporting, reviewing and acting upon errors and near misses. The so-called 'untoward events' that have always formed part of clinical practice must now be used to learn and thereby to enable the protection of future patients. This is part and parcel of the risk management process and should mean an increased and earlier awareness of mistakes and problems with management.

Studies from around the world (Localio *et al.* 1991) suggest that 4–7% of all hospital admissions suffer from something going wrong, a so-called 'untoward event'. Not all of these are serious or have grave consequences but this is none the less a high percentage of mistakes. It is crucial to realize that there is seldom one individual at fault when something goes wrong. More commonly, mistakes occur as a consequence of a series of errors, mishaps and administrative acts. Despite increased pressure for openness and honesty and efforts towards the existence of a 'no blame culture', doctors feel that they are expected to function without error. Thus when mistakes occur they may feel isolated in their response to this and unable to talk it through with their colleagues.

It is essential in this climate of scrutiny, league tables and reporting pressure that doctors accept that mistakes are an inevitable part of practice, which often have system errors as their root cause—inadequate staffing and resources, poor supervision in training and long hours all play their part. A climate of openness and honesty in reporting such mistakes for analysis and lessons to be learned is necessary and this must run in tandem with the maturity and compassion to discuss what has occurred fully and freely with the interested party—the patient.

On the other side of the coin, however, is the tendency, where a patient experiences an unexpected adverse outcome, for the concerned clinician to accept fault where there is none. There may be a variety of reasons for this. A feeling that the patient has in someway been 'short-changed' by a system with long waiting lists and inadequate time for full explanations and assessments; a system that also does not allow for proper training and supervision of juniors. The guilt may arise because the task has been delegated to a doctor in training and the senior doctor feels that he should have performed it personally.

When things go wrong

The desire to help is often the driving force behind a decision to enter clinical practice. When things go wrong in medicine it is not only the patient who suffers. There is huge attrition and sadness on the part of the clinicians. Many may question their continuance of practice fearing that they will not be able to forget the error that they made.

There have been enormous developments in the field of clinical practice over recent decades. There is great media interest in all matters medical and the Internet provides access to detailed information on any aspect of care to all. All of this means that many patients may now be extremely knowledgeable about their treatment options and expectations run high.

Many say that anger is at the heart of all medical negligence litigation. It is appropriate to feel concerned and anxious when treatment does not go according to plan. There is a fine line between anger and anxiety and the fear of what complications may arise can act as a catalyst to change an anxious and afraid patient into an angry one. Where the patient is 'kept in the dark' and feels in any way isolated, this is a recipe for disaster. In the words of Lady Macbeth 'present fears are less than horrible imaginings'. A patient who has had an unexpected outcome, which is unsatisfactory, if left to brood will swiftly become angry and resentful. Often anger can be defused if there is prompt recognition of a problem and an explanation of what has happened and what can be done to improve the outcome.

When faced with an angry, distressed patient it is essential to let that patient have his say and talk about his problem. Meeting anger with anger is a disaster. Instead, the patient deserves an analysis of what has caused the anger, a sympathetic explanation of what has happened and the options that are available. If the treating clinician has to involve a colleague to improve the outcome, this should be done at the earliest possible opportunity. In this way the harm to the patient is minimized. This is of duel benefit; it is morally right to improve a poor outcome and this may in turn protect the clinical relationship so that the doctor feels able to continue to treat the patient. An additional benefit relates to the level of compensation should a claim in negligence follow, the damages payable will reflect the speed of resolution of the problem. (See below, Liability.)

What underpins successful and fulfilled clinical practice is the relationship with patients. No relationship can survive in the absence of honesty. It is a common courtesy to extend an explanation to any individual to whom one owes a duty of care where the outcome is not satisfactory. It is not only rude to avoid angry or upset patients it is also the surest way to press them towards a complaint or litigation.

As has already been indicated, many may feel that saying sorry constitutes an admission of liability. A sincere and honest apology is a proper expression of regret to any patient who has suffered a misfortune. Apologizing that such an event should have occurred is a courtesy, which should not be confused with a formal admission of legal liability. In this respect it is not prudent to ask the treating clinician to offer an impartial view of his or his team's treatment of a patient. The treating clinician is all too often 'too close to the woods to see the trees'. Additionally pressure is often felt, by the clinician in charge to offer an immediate commentary together with an explanation and an apology, regardless of whether the full facts are to hand. It is important to take sufficient time to discover exactly what the sequence was so that the information given to the patient is a true and accurate reflection of the facts. Bear in mind the adage 'speak in haste and repent at leisure'. Trying to maintain the patient's trust where there is an inaccuracy, which inevitably comes to light, is a problem best avoided particularly against a background of anxiety and concern.

The issue of liability should be kept separate from the immediate events and their consequences. This more often than not requires a view from a colleague who is also expert in the field who is entirely independent of the issues and as such does not allow his judgement to be clouded by the regret of an unhappy outcome for his patient. Telling the patient or relative that this is the planned course of action can help to provide the needed reassurance that no one is trying to create the oft heralded 'conspiracy of silence' or the medical 'cover-up'.

What do patients want when things go wrong?

An apology—'No one ever said they were sorry even though we had been through a terrible time'

An explanation and answers to questions—'I wanted to know what had happened and why'

Accountability—'No one should have to be treated as I was. I want justice. Heads should roll. He should be struck off'

Help—'I wanted my mum to have more help. Before all this she was really independent. She lost confidence and could have really been helped if someone had come even for a short each day until the stitches were healed'

Change—'I want to know that systems have been changed and that lessons have been learned'

Communication with patients

The clinical relationship, in common with all relationships, relies on the two-way process of listening and speaking. It is essential to remember not only the nature of what is to be said to the patient but also the manner in which it is delivered. This is never more true than when the information to be shared is bad news.

A great deal of the rapport with patients depends on open and accurate communication. It is important therefore to ensure that the facts are to hand when having a full and definitive discussion of events. This should not stop the clinician approaching the patient early on in the sequence simply to say that enquiries are being made and that a full explanation and discussion will take place as soon as the facts are known. A defensive, arrogant or dismissive attitude from the clinician spells disaster for all parties.

The discussion, which eventually takes places with the facts to hand, should be conducted by a senior member of the team. While junior staff may be encouraged to sit in on the discussion (where appropriate) this is not the time for the old adage of 'see one, do one, teach one'. The patient should not be suddenly placed alone in a situation of vulnerability where, with no prior warning, he is suddenly confronted with a barrage of facts and proposals about his treatment to date and as planned. This is a situation where the patient should have the opportunity to have a close family member or friend with him for moral support, to act as an extra pair of ears and to ask pertinent questions on his behalf.

This meeting should be in circumstances, which are conducive to information sharing. The location should ideally be comfortable and private. This conversation is not one for a bedside with flimsy curtains hiding nothing in the presence of a large and daunting entourage. Nor should this conversation be 'squeezed in' to a pressured outpatient scenario with 5 minutes per consultation.

Verbal and listening skills

Having said that the patient must have a chance to 'let off steam', so-called 'active listening' can help. Asking questions or offering non-verbal support cues can emphasize that you are listening. Interruptions should be avoided as they may imply a wish to control or manipulate the discussion. It is important to establish and maintain patient confidence in the face of a difficult situation for both parties. Eye contact helps to emphasize empathy, as does body language. Lack of eye contact can be interpreted as embarrassment or dishonesty. There is no place for a rushed explanation laded with technical jargon. Speech, which is slow, clear and comprehensible, is essential. Frequent pauses give the patient an opportunity to ask questions and to seek clarification of points.

Bearing in mind that few patients retain more that a third of what has been imparted in any clinical interview, it is helpful to give an opportunity for a further meeting after a period of digestion of the facts. A brief summary or overview at the end of the meeting can also help.

Saying sorry!

Speedy—speak to the patient as soon as possible/with facts to hand

Open—honesty is essential

Relevant—simple non-technical language helps

Responsive—where possible steps to minimize harm should be taken

Yours—ownership is important/'passing the buck' does not help anyone

Liability

As has already been canvassed, many concerns expressed about apologizing relate to the concern that in expressing regret, there is a tacit acceptance of fault and therefore an admission of liability. Doctors fear that by offering an apology or expression of regret they open the floodgates to a legal claim.

It is important to be aware that funding claims, where there is medical negligence comes from two major sources: the Defence Bodies (the Medical Protection Society, the Medical and Dental Defence Union of Scotland and the Medical Defence Union) and the National Health Service Litigation Authority (NHSLA). The Defence Bodies provide indemnity for GPs and private practitioners and the NHSLA fund negligence claims against NHS Trusts. Both bodies are quite clear that patients who suffer harm are entitled to a full and frank explanation and an apology. Dr Kathleen Allsopp from

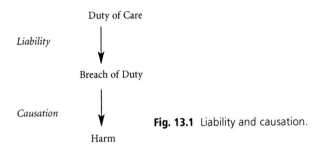

Fig. 13.1 Liability and causation.

the Medical Defence Union stated that defence body's view back in 1986 and this view has since been confirmed by the NHSLA.

The UK courts judge liability on the basis of what is considered to be acceptable by a body of 'medical men skilled in that art'. In order to qualify for financial compensation, the patient/claimant must be able to show that the defendant doctor owed him a duty of care and that the care offered fell below an acceptable level. This is the liability aspect of any claim. Thereafter, in order to assess the damages payable it is necessary to assess the harm that flowed, as a consequence of this breach of duty. This is the causation side of the equation. In order to receive compensation the claimant must be able to demonstrate that harm flowed as a direct consequence of the breach of duty (see Fig. 13.1).

Confidentiality

Family

Many of the difficult conversations in clinical practice take place with the patient's relatives. It is essential to be mindful of the duty of confidentiality. Often faced with a difficult situation and an unexpectedly poor outcome the clinician may seek to explain what has occurred to relatives feeling that this is in the patient's best interests and what the patient may want. First and foremost the duty is to the patient and the clinical duty carries with it the burden of confidentiality. Better therefore to have such frank and open discussions in the presence of the patient or with his full consent to the disclosure of information to close family.

Media

It is also essential to be mindful of this duty where an incident attracts the attention of the local media. An approach by a journalist for comments does not provide 'carte blanche' for that patient and his experiences to be disclosed to the paper without the patient's full knowledge and consent.

Summary

1. Where a patient has suffered harm, regardless of fault or the potential for litigation they deserve a full explanation and an apology.

2. An apology is extended as an expression of sympathy and is not a legal admission of liability. It is not appropriate for the treating clinical team to be drawn into

complex legal liability issues. These are better dealt with by those more distant from the treating sequence who are able to be impartial in offering judgements.

3. Every effort should be made for discussions to be fully informed.

4. Time should be taken to ascertain the correct facts before wading in with half-baked explanations.

5. Investigations should be thorough and prompt.

6. It is essential that senior staff carry out the discussions with the patient, although the juniors should be involved in the process as much as possible.

7. The patient should be given the opportunity to have a companion present for any discussion.

8. Having had a full, frank and detailed discussion with the patient, it is sensible while the facts are fresh to make a note of what was said by the various parties.

9. The discussion should take place in a situation where there is privacy and time.

10. It is important to speak clearly and allow plenty of time for questions and the opportunity for a further meeting.

11. Arrangements to support the patient and ameliorate the condition should be put in hand swiftly. Harmed patients deserve 'Rolls Royce' treatment from the health service.

12. Providing factual information and proposals for future management assists in the explanatory process.

13. It is essential to be aware that having been involved in a clinical incident where a patient is harmed, the clinician *and* the patient require support.

Case studies

Case 1

On 19 February 2001, a 6-year-old child had surgery for a convergent squint. At the end of the operation the swab count was noted to be incomplete. The senior registrar in ophthalmology who had performed the operation attended the child and her mother after the child had returned to the ward and explained what had happened but also that he was sure that the swab had fallen to the ground during the procedure and a full check had been made to ensure that the swab was not in the eye.

Postoperatively the child had a number of problems with eye symptoms. These were similar to problems, which she had had in the past, and on no occasion was anything found by the examining doctor. She developed a subconjunctival cyst and this was removed under a general anaesthetic.

On 5 March 2002, 13 months after the original procedure, the child's mother telephoned the hospital to say that she had a swab which had come out of her daughter's eye and that there was a lot of pus. The consultant, who was in overall charge, saw her 2 days later. She was well with no eye symptoms. He was shown the swab. It was an eye swab in good condition. The notes were not to hand at this time.

The consultant offered an immediate and frank apology to the mother. He wrote to the GP to confirm that he had seen the swab and it was the type of swab used in eye surgery. He said that he would report this as an untoward incident and recommend that lessons be implemented by the use of a new design of swab so that this could not happen again.

A letter of complaint was received from the mother on 10 March. She indicated that she considered that her daughter has suffered unacceptable pain and discomfort and that she was angry that this had happened and would be seeking compensation on her behalf. The letter and the notes were passed to the consultant eye surgeon. He then confirmed the following:

- He had read the notes made by the operating surgeon who detailed the efforts made to locate the swab, which had been seen falling on to the surgical drapes.
- Additionally he confirmed that he had personally examined the child's eye on several occasions and it was inconceivable that he could have failed to see a swab.
- He confirmed that the size of the swab was such that it would have created an obvious swelling, which would have abraded the eyelid and been intolerably painful.
- In his view there was no possibility that this swab could have been left in place for the period alleged.

A letter was sent from the Trust to the child's mother, explaining that it was difficult to explain how the swab could have been retained and she was asked if the swab could be examined forensically. A solicitor's letter followed suggesting that liability and causation could not be denied and the Trust was urged to make settlement proposals.

Instead a detailed letter outlining the sequence of events and the surgeon's comments was sent to the solicitors who were urged to review the merits of this case. A letter was received shortly after from the solicitors to indicate that they would not be proceeding with the claim.

Lessons

In the circumstances of the facts as presented, the consultant surgeon sought to offer a full and frank apology. He made himself personally available within 48 hours to meet with the mother and to see the child. He sought to reassure the mother as to the long-term sequelae and also took steps to protect future patients. He did not have the notes to hand and was thus not fully apprised of the facts and the underlying picture. Nor did he take full heed of the size of the swab in question and thus the impracticality of the allegation.

This then was a good, careful and caring clinician seeking to offer an apology and make amends. The outcome was a letter of complaint and swift recourse to solicitors.

While one cannot expect that complaints and allegations will usually be entirely spurious, it is always prudent to take whatever steps are possible to be fully aware of the sequence of events before going into detail beyond expressing sympathy at the concerns being voiced.

Case 2

A 40-year-old man presented to the Accident and Emergency department. He was anxious and had severe chest pain. He was a poor historian and had a history of previous alcohol abuse. A provisional diagnosis of gastritis was made and he was allowed home after 2 hours as the pain had settled.

He remained unwell at home and re-presented to his GP a week later. He said that he had been feeling dreadful all week but had hesitated to trouble another doctor after his experience in A&E. The GP had concerns that he might have pneumonia or pleurisy and he was sent back to the hospital. On this occasion he was admitted. The diagnosis proved difficult and it was a further week before it became apparent that he had a spontaneous splenic rupture for which a splenectomy was undertaken. He had a stormy postoperative course but eventually made a full recovery and was discharged.

There was no letter of complaint or mention of any dissatisfaction but a letter was received from solicitors seeking access to the records and alleging that the splenectomy had been performed without proper informed consent.

A detailed review of the notes revealed them to be in a very poor state. They were disorganized and many entries were difficult to read and incomplete in the information they contained. The comments of the clinical staff made it clear that the signs with which the patient presented were difficult to interpret and the ultimate diagnosis was extremely rare. It was felt that the claim would not succeed and in due course confirmation was received from the solicitors that this was indeed the case.

A telephone interview was conducted by the Trust's medico-legal adviser at the conclusion of this claim in order to seek to understand what had provoked it. It transpired that:

- The patient felt really unwell when he attended A&E but was made to feel as if he were 'making a fuss'.
- He had not felt well enough to be sent home but rather that they were effectively throwing him out.
- At home he continued to feel really ill but was too scared to go to his GP or back to the Trust after his earlier treatment.
- When he did see his GP he was obviously concerned about what he found and sent him into hospital.
- In hospital no one really explained anything. He continued to feel worse and worse and no one seemed to be doing anything.
- Things then suddenly got much worse and he ended up having a big operation and not really knowing why.

Lessons

This was an entirely avoidable claim. The patient sought legal advice against a background of anger and lack of understanding. He felt that his treatment had been poor because no one ever told him what was happening or why. While there were no actual costs borne by the hospital there were the administrative costs of photocopying a large volume of records for disclosure and the time taken by several senior staff to review the notes and offer comments on liability and causation.

The solicitor dealing with the case was pleased and surprised to be contacted by the Trust's representative at the conclusion of the case. He felt it helpful to have a chance to express his client's concerns and was pleased to be able to relay to him that the Trust regretted that he had felt the need to resort to litigation.

Case 3

A 26-year-old housewife attended her local hospital for the shared care of her first pregnancy. She had a normal delivery of a healthy baby boy in June 2000. She had sustained a first-degree tear and this was sutured by the locum registrar, who had supervised the delivery.

She was discharged home after 2 days and was attended by the community midwife in the usual way. She complained of some perineal and abdominal pain and was reassured that this was 'normal in new mums'.

She was concerned that she smelt bad and even her husband commented that he found it hard to be in the same room as her. Twelve days after the birth, when sitting in the bath she pulled out a long tailed vaginal swab. This had been inserted while the episiotomy was sutured and left there. It was extremely offensive.

She was angry and horrified and phoned the hospital the next day. She was seen by the consultant in charge of her care and he apologized for what she had experienced. He undertook to contact the doctor who had left the swab *in situ* and to tell her what transpired.

Fortunately the patient made a full recovery after a short course of antibiotics. She did not, however, hear further from the Trust. The locum could not be traced and this case thus 'slipped through the net'. There was no notification of an untoward incident and thus no opportunity for the Trust to act proactively with the patient.

The next event was a letter of claim from solicitors. They sought £10 000 in compensation and alleged that not only had their client suffered immediate discomfort but she had also had problems bonding with her baby and probably would not be able to contemplate any more children.

A swift investigation of events led to the conclusion that the claim was indefensible but that the sum sought was excessive. A more realistic sum was subsequently agreed and funded by the NHSLA. In addition to the payment the patient asked that she be sent a formal letter of apology from the chief executive. This was duly done.

Lessons

This claim illustrates the need for timely investigation and apologies as well as the use of the reporting framework so that lessons are learned and shared. An early, sympathetic and frank apology is likely to have avoided the need for litigation. It would have remained open to the patient to say that she felt that compensation was due to her and this is something that the Trust could have negotiated with her direct. She would have been advised in these circumstances that it was open to her to approach solicitors and their costs would be met. Many patients are happy to negotiate direct with the Trust knowing that every effort will be made to ensure that they are fairly compensated.

The case also illustrates the problems attendant on the use of locum staff. With no ongoing commitment to the Trust or Practice, locums commonly do not respond to letters seeking comments on complaints or untoward events, which occurred during their period of employment. If this is to change, a more secure method of reliably contacting such personnel has to be established.

References

A Fish called Wanda (1988). Paramount Pictures.

Brazier, M. (1992). *Medicine Patients and the Law.* London: Penguin Books.

Confidentiality: Protecting and Providing Information (2000). *General Medical Council Publications.* London: GMC.

Good Medical Practice (1998). *General Medical Council Publications.* London: GMC.

Hiatt, H.H., Barnes, B.A., Brennan, T.A., *et al.* (1989). A study of medical history and medical malpractice. *New England Journal of Medicine*, 1989; **312**, 480–4.

John, Elton. *Sorry Seems to Be the Hardest Word.*

Journal of the Medical Defence Union (1986). Spring 1986, **2**(2), 2.

Localio, A.R., Lawthers, A.G., Brennan, T.A., *et al.* (1991). Relation between malpractice claims and adverse events due to negligence: results of the Harvard medical practice study 111. *New England Journal of Medicine*, **325**, 245–51.

Making Amends (2003). Clinical Negligence Reform—Department of Health UK 2003 Consultation paper, www.dh.gov.uk.

Mason, J.K. and McCall Smith, R.A. (1994). *Law and Medical Ethics.* Oxford: Butterworths.

Mulcahy, L., Lloyd, S. (1999). *Medical Mishaps—Pieces of the Puzzle.* Bostock: Open University Press.

Vincent, C. (2001). *Clinical Risk Management.* London: BMJ Books.

Chapter 14

Legal constraints and guidelines to good practice

Liz Martinez

Summary

This chapter approaches the subject of doctor–patient communication from the perspective of a lawyer with over a decade of experience in handling medical negligence claims on behalf of patients. Practical advice on communication is offered with the intention of avoiding the need for patients to resort to litigation in order to meet their needs for information, explanations and apologies when their medical treatment fails to meet their expectations.

Society's expectations: 'not just Bristol'

In 1996 The Right Honourable Lord Woolf, Master of the Rolls, undertook a review of the civil justice system, which brought about a complete overhaul in the way civil legal cases are managed by the court. In his report, *Access to Justice*, he identified medical negligence litigation as the area most in need of change. He emphasized the extent of the mistrust between claimants and defendants (i.e. patient and doctor/health-care provider NHS Trust) and made a series of recommendations that included the suggestion that doctors be obliged to communicate to their patient when mistakes have happened in their care (in the same way, for example, that solicitors are obliged to tell a client to seek alternative advice when they have acted inappropriately). The objective was to achieve more openness within the doctor–patient relationship with a view to reducing the role of litigation to the last resort.

> 'The suspicion between the parties is intense and the lack of co-operation frequently greater than in many other areas of litigation …'
> 'The cause for concern is the amount of money spent by NHS Trusts and other defendants on legal costs: money which would be much better devoted to compensating victims or, better still, to improving standards of care so that future mistakes are avoided …'
> 'Many people involved in medical negligence litigation have justifiably pointed out to me the importance of establishing from the outset what an injured patient wants. Proceedings often start because the claimant cannot get the information he is seeking, or an explanation or apology, from the doctor or hospital. Historically, solicitors have had no alternative but to advise legal action, which is unlikely to be appropriate in all cases unless the client's main or only objective is to obtain financial compensation …'
> 'The best way of dealing with the problem of delay before claims are started would be a policy of more open communication on the part of hospital staff …'
>
> Selected extracts, Woolf (1996)

Mediation (a form of alternative dispute resolution or ADR) was also recommended as an excellent way of dealing with difficult and entrenched disputes that are threatening to get to court, and indeed it is very effective. Should it really be necessary, however, for there to be an intermediary in order to achieve communication between doctor and patient? Wouldn't it be simpler, cheaper and more rewarding for all concerned to avoid the need for dispute resolution altogether by the use of good communication and mediation skills in general everyday interactions with patients, in the course of their normal working relationship?

Dispelling the myth

My experience from speaking to groups of doctors, at all levels, but particularly to junior doctors, is that there is a perceived threat of litigation from patients thought to have unrealistically high expectations, which is ever present in the mind of today's doctor.

It is true that clinical negligence litigation is on the increase. Patients are more aware of their rights and may seek the advice of a solicitor following medical care, which they believe to have been unsatisfactory. In my experience as a claimants' solicitor in a legal practice, the majority of patients who seek legal advice are advised not to proceed with a claim through the court once their concerns have been investigated properly. The advice not to proceed may follow a limited investigation in which a request is made for medical records to be disclosed and a report is obtained from an independent medical expert who advises that the treatment was in accordance with accepted standards. Alternatively, the patient may be discouraged from proceeding at the first meeting with the solicitor when the patient is told about the law and the very strict circumstances in which a clinical negligence claim may be investigated and pursued. It should therefore be of reassurance to doctors to understand that unless treatment falls far below generally accepted standards of care it is very hard for a patient to succeed with a claim in negligence.

In summary, the patient is advised that in order for us to establish that a doctor has been negligent we must prove that no other reasonable body of competent medical opinion would condone the treatment that was given. The mere fact that another medical practitioner might have acted differently is not enough to prove that the doctor or medical team in your case was negligent as long as they have acted in a way that accords with generally acceptable standards. This is known as the Bolam test (from a legal case *Bolam v Friern Hospital Management Committee 1957*) and is used as the starting point to determine whether medical treatment given to a patient was negligent. The Bolam test must be satisfied for any case in negligence to succeed.

Other case law has determined that doctors are allowed (and expected) to exercise clinical judgement, but the standard of care is objective, and is not reduced if the care happens to be administered by an inexperienced doctor.

Once negligence has been established that is not the end of the story for the patient. It must also be proven that the particular negligent act or omission has caused significant damage to the patient (causation), and it is the assessment of the damage that has been directly caused by the negligence (physical, certain types of psychological damage, and certain types of financial loss) that gives rise to the claim for compensation. Without causation of significant damage there is no justification for proceeding with a legal claim, even if there has been negligence on the part of the doctor.

The only remedy that a court can order in such a claim is compensation. The court cannot order that the patient be given an explanation or apology, or that systems be changed to prevent the same mistake from happening again, and yet, often, that is all that the patient really wanted.

Litigation should be the last resort

There are so many opportunities for communication prior to the patient instructing a solicitor that it should be rare for patients to need the services of a solicitor unless compensation is needed in cases of severe injury with consequent ongoing disability or financial loss.

There are doctor–patient interactions before treatment, during treatment (unless the patient is unconscious), (immediately) after treatment, and often at follow-up appointments.

If a patient makes a complaint orally or expresses concerns about treatment then ideally, the best time to address it is immediately. This may not always be possible. If it is necessary to defer discussing the complaint then make a special appointment to discuss it soon and keep to the appointment. Be familiar with the NHS Complaints Procedure and actively support the local resolution process while the patient is still interested in dialogue with you or the hospital. At this early stage responsiveness, openness and willingness to listen and address the patient's key concerns are vital if the patient is to feel satisfied.

If no resolution has been reached by this time there are likely to be intermediaries or advocates involved such as client advocates from the Community Health Councils (CHCs)/Patient Advice and Liaison Service, lawyers, and the health-care provider's own team of complaints officers and risk managers. From now on open communication is discouraged, filtered through legal and risk management strategy and perspectives and delayed by bureaucracy. At no time from now on will there be the opportunity to communicate one to one, person to person unless some forward thinking lawyers for both parties advise mediation. You have lost control of the process, which now becomes protracted, expensive, geared towards compensation and extremely worrying for doctor and patient alike. You can expect the litigation process to last up to 3 years.

What do patients want?

When considering the need for enhanced and conscious communication training I would encourage doctors to adopt a change of mindset. Compensation claims are not bad. Poor medical practice is bad. We are not simply trying to avoid litigation for compensation. The patient has a right to be compensated for personal injury caused by negligence, just as you might claim on another driver's insurance when that driver has damaged your car negligently. Rather we want to increase awareness as to the reason why patients choose to litigate in order to improve medical practice by improving communication.

From my experience, when patients consult a solicitor about investigating their treatment with a view to a claim they:

- ◆ Feel aggrieved by medical treatment.
- ◆ May be injured, or someone they love may be injured.
- ◆ May have had a relative die.
- ◆ May be confused, angry, shocked, traumatized, or upset about what has happened to them.
- ◆ May just want to know—'an explanation'.

They consult a solicitor at various stages:

- ◆ Immediately after treatment (I find this the saddest. If there has been no attempt to communicate I try to encourage the patient to go back and ask for an explanation).
- ◆ After the impact of the injury has begun to sink in and they are starting to question their treatment.
- ◆ After attempts to get information have failed, including at complaints procedure.
- ◆ More rarely after an apology or formal admission of liability has been made and they are seeking advice about appropriate levels of compensation. At this stage the patient may even have been advised to see a specialist solicitor by the health-care provider.

What do patients want when they consult a solicitor about medical treatment?

Accountability

They want to know who is to blame, who has inflicted this injury upon them or a loved one. Accountability of this kind is difficult to establish in the NHS where the system takes responsibility for the errors of individuals, and where admissions of liability are rarely offered.

There may also be underlying factors, such as fear or guilt, as frequently seen in cases involving disabled children, where the patient or parent needs to be reassured that the injury or disability is not their fault.

I have found it interesting to note how many times a patient seeks to attach the blame to the wrong person in a medical team when another wonderful doctor is discovered on investigation actually to have been responsible for the negligent act. I would suggest that this arises from the misconception that the best communicator was the better doctor.

Apology (see Chapter 13)

Patients want the common courtesy of a timely apology from the person who made the mistake or caused the injury, in the same way that after accidentally stepping on their foot you would apologize straight away.

The best some patients get is a weak, embarrassed expression of sympathy or apology from the defendant Trust's barrister after a heavily contested court case. Even after winning their case some patients don't feel satisfied until they have a written letter of apology.

Explanation

They want an explanation from an appropriate person, who is usually the same person they have seen before, or someone they trust giving them the explanation first hand.

On many occasions I have seen how a badly written response to a complaint can aggravate rather than ameliorate the patient's desire to seek legal redress. Such letters are written by a third party, dismissive of the patient's own concerns, and often inaccurate on further scrutiny.

Altruism

In many cases the patient may simply need to know that what has happened to them will not happen to anyone else, particularly after treatment has led to someone's death, or if they have survived a very shocking or unpleasant experience. In such cases they are not interested in the paltry level of compensation that is attributable to the death of someone with no dependants (e.g. the elderly or a child). They want to see evidence that someone has learned from their experience. They are very highly aggravated by hearing of other similar events in the same hospital or by the same doctor. If changes are promised through a complaints procedure, adverse event reporting or are recommended by an independent review panel or a coroner, the patient may want to see evidence of the change, or may appreciate a letter advising them that as a result of their experience changes have been made.

Compensation

As discussed above, compensation is an entitlement for personal injury caused by negligent health care. Many patients want to be compensated for their injury or loss. In the absence of accountability, apology or evidence of learning from the mistake, compensation is the only available form of redress.

Compensation may be needed for care, or to make up financial losses arising from injury. Very little compensation is awarded when it can't make a difference to the patient, for example after death of a child or where a past or future financial loss arising directly from the negligent act cannot be proven.

Litigation

At some stage in a first interview with a new client they will usually ask for reassurance from the solicitor that they won't need to go to court. In my experience litigation is rarely a positive desire of the aggrieved patient. It may be seen as the only option to obtain one of the other remedies already discussed or a way to ensure that the health-care provider takes notice of their complaint. Litigation is costly, time consuming, a last resort that provides at best an artificial 'truth', and rarely addresses all of the patient's real concerns.

A complaint will not necessarily end in litigation, but regardless of whether or not a patient's complaint ends up in court the process is costly, distracting, stressful, and embarrassing. The best way to avoid it is by good communication.

Occasionally, there are people who wish to abuse the system, to seek financial gain where this is not justified (just as occasionally there are doctors who for various reasons do not have the motivations or behaviours that we expect of our health-care providers). In my experience these people are rare, and the combination of the legal framework within which claims are made and the ethical standards of lawyers discourage such people from succeeding with their claims.

A brief word about criminal/disciplinary proceedings

Civil (negligence/compensation) litigation will not usually result in criminal, or disciplinary proceedings or striking off unless the action is very serious indeed and constitutes a criminal offence or breaches professional codes of conduct. This book does not purport to advise doctors as to criminal or disciplinary matters.

The medical records may be inspected by patients, their lawyers, the doctor's own lawyers, or the coroner, after a patient makes a complaint. It may be a criminal offence to alter medical records, which may be regarded as evidence for the court. Following an inquest in which I represented a client a few years ago the Coroner reported the NHS Trust to the Director of Public Prosecutions to consider whether there were grounds for a charge of conspiracy to pervert the course of justice after the records had been altered. There are strict procedures for altering medical records both in the case of the patient's request to do so and on the part of the doctor. If you need to add to records in any way you must seek legal advice before doing so and in any event you should only make additional notes on a separate piece of paper, which is dated (at the date of alteration) and signed, and the reason for the late addition should be noted.

Invasive medical treatment without consent is an assault and may also be a criminal offence. There are limited exceptions to this rule, for example where treatment is given without consent pursuant to a court order or where the patient is a child (in which case parental consent should be sought and the doctor should act in the best interests of the patient), or where they are mentally incapable of giving consent.

In certain circumstances inhumane or degrading medical treatment is now a breach of Article 3 of the Human Rights Act 1998.

Practical recommendations for good communication

Before, during and immediately after treatment

- When giving difficult advice be 'stunningly straight' then deal with the consequences. I picked up this valuable advice from a high-powered business woman who was speaking at a seminar I attended a few years ago. It is true for this situation.

- Tell the whole truth. A full explanation has value rather than confuses. In a set of medical records I was once reading I came across a letter from a paediatrician to the obstetrician following a difficult shoulder dystocia case resulting in Erb's palsy. The paediatrician had been asked to explain what had happened at the birth. The explanation, according to the paediatrician, had been as follows: 'Father asked about the obstetric side. I told him that once one had delivered the head one was obliged to deliver the body.' Litigation inevitably followed.

- Be aware of and compliant with confidentiality restraints when talking to relatives.

- Remember that people instinctively know when something is wrong or when they are not being told the truth (or something is being hidden from them). In neurolinguistic programming* it is called 'congruence'. You communicate with the whole person. This is not about body language tricks. It is about being open, honest and secure enough to communicate fully with the patient and their family if necessary.

- Patients want to hear difficult information from the right person, someone they know and trust, someone with the relevant knowledge. If the right person has delegated this task to you, be sure that you are well informed and that you introduce yourself to the patient and let them know that you are fully aware of their circumstances.

- Patients believe that good communicators are the best doctors. Be a good communicator.

- Do not assume your patient is unintelligent or incapable of hearing the truth, especially when they ask for it! The truth may hurt but it is less hurtful than discovering that you have been misled or kept in the dark about very important and personal matters. Why should an inarticulate or less-educated or non-professional person be entitled to less information?

- Adapt how you tell them the information rather than what you say.

- The timing of explanations is important. Patients occasionally report that they have been given an explanation when they were trying to come round from an anaesthetic and did not understand or retain a word of it. Equally, patients don't want to wait for days for an explanation. This is a balancing act. Explanations should be given as soon as they are capable of taking in the information (e.g. that the operation did not go as planned) allowing for further opportunities to ask questions at a later stage if necessary.

----

* NLP or neurolinguistic programming is a personal developmental tool in which one uses language, rapport skills and various mental tricks to enhance communication and performance and as a very powerful form of therapy.

Warnings and consent

- Warn of risks properly, clearly and honestly. Be aware of the law and guidance with regard to consent. Dissatisfaction can be thought of as the gap between expectation and outcome. Don't be ambiguous or untruthful in order to steer the patient towards the recommended treatment. The patient is entitled to be informed and to make his own choice.

- Avoid sound bites and inaccurate clichés. A patient who had suffered injury to her ureter in a hysterectomy operation told me: 'He told me I would be a new woman after the hysterectomy'. She was. She was incontinent. An expert in the litigation summed up the effect of the consenting procedure: 'She may well have been warned of the risks but generally left the consultant's room with a feeling of optimism about the treatment she was about to receive. It will change her life'.

- Remember that patients are human, responsible, entitled to make their own decisions (even illogical or unusual decisions) about their own treatment unless they are mentally incapable of giving consent (see law of consent). The mere fact that they make an illogical decision does not render them mentally incompetent. They have legally enforceable human rights and are entitled to be treated with respect and dignity.

- The timing of taking informed consent from a patient is important. Poor timing may invalidate the patient's ability to give consent, for example seeking consent for a sterilization when the patient is on the way down to theatre for a caesarean section.

Records

- Record accurately what you tell the patient.

- Be aware of the Data Protection Act 1998, which gives the patient the right to disclosure of their medical records. Accurate recording will provide protection for you (assuming you have acted competently) when justifying warnings given, treatment refused, etc. Allow for the fact that you will have forgotten the detail of this interaction in 3 years time if a case goes to court. The patient probably won't as it is of great importance to them. Your records are your memory.

- Remember that when patients exercise their right to see their records they should not read for the first time the truth about their illness, prognosis, etc. At its worst a clear discrepancy between advice given orally to patients and their family and what is recorded in the medical notes can be an abuse. An obvious and frequent example is where the elderly mentally competent patient's records are marked in code to show that the patient is not for resuscitation when this has not been discussed with the patient or the family.

- Remember that in court good note taking suggests good doctoring!

- And vice versa. This is an extract from a genuine letter in some medical records I read some years ago: 'Dear doctor, this gentleman's notes were not available. I do not know what operation he has had. Anyway he is getting better and I would like to see him in the clinic in 2 months.'

Some ethical issues (see Chapter 3 for a full discussion of ethics)

- Realize that your own discomfort or fears will affect how you communicate with a patient. Can you sit with the patient's discomfort about bad news or pain and not feel the need to avoid the truth in order to fix it? It is very difficult to do and yet essential for the doctor in learning to communicate with patients in difficult situations. Compassion and genuine efforts to help are different from 'care-taking' in which you attempt to minimize or dismiss the real problem. You may get inappropriately involved with the patient to help yourself handle the emotions that the patient's care brings up for you rather than retaining an appropriate doctor–patient relationship. Be clear with yourself about your own feelings, fears and doubts and if necessary (and possible) seek supervision before going into the meeting with the patient.

- Don't feel obliged to advise in areas outside your expertise. You will be regarded as all-knowledgeable and professional and have direct influence over patients who are vulnerable.

A full discussion of the ethical issues involved in caring can be found in The Ethics of Caring (1995), Taylor, K. Hanford Mead.

Immediate action

If something goes wrong deal with it immediately (see Chapter 13 on Clinical risk management and governance). Write up a summary of the events immediately, date and sign it. Discuss your concerns with appropriate colleagues and obtain emotional support. See what can be done to help the patient, or to minimize the damage to the patient. Realize that everyone makes mistakes. Your integrity and your reputation lie in the way in which you deal with them.

Communication after the event

- Say sorry early (see apology above and Chapter 13). Learn the difference between a genuine human apology and a legal admission of liability!

- Remember that good doctors can make mistakes. Bad doctors cover them up, fail to learn from them and perpetuate the problem in order to avoid taking responsibility. Suspected cover up almost guarantees the patients will seek legal advice.

- Equality of power will affect the dynamic of the communication. Many patients feel intimidated by doctors, however educated they may be, when the interaction concerns their own illness and vulnerability. They may also feel overwhelmed or intimidated when expected to discuss their concerns about their treatment in a room filled with the treating doctor, his consultant, the chief executive of the Trust, a complaints officer and someone else there taking the minutes of the meeting. This is often how complaints procedure 'local resolution' meetings are conducted. The mind goes blank in the presence of the doctor concerned and they forget to ask the questions they wanted to or are unable to express them clearly. Encourage them to write questions down beforehand and bring them with them so that you can answer them. Allow them to bring a friend, or a CHC representative or Patient Advice and Liaison Service representative with them. Allow them time to take notes if they want to so that they can remember and think about what you have said. They may need an opportunity to revisit or ask follow-up questions.

+ The relevant issues will not be the same for each party. You may need to elicit carefully from the patient what they are really concerned about as they may not express these concerns directly or clearly. It is essential to address the *patient's* key concern however irrelevant it may seem if you want the patient to be satisfied. Mediation is a good forum for eliciting and addressing these hidden but essential keys to resolution, but mediation skills can be used in any situation. What is relevant differs with perspective and with context. Prior to treatment it is essential that the *doctor's* relevant issues (e.g. warnings of risks, likely outcomes, side-effects) are clearly emphasized, and the patient has the chance to ask questions afterwards, discuss and assimilate what he has heard. Ideally the doctor should then summarize again the key points if possible. While the patient was thinking of their question they may not have been listening carefully to the advice that was given. Get the patient to repeat the key points if you don't think they have understood.

Finally

There has been a great deal of discussion about talking to patients. However, good communication is two-way and interactive. As professionals employed to be knowledgeable and advise we often forget that a major key to communication is to listen. In many of the legal cases that I have seen the patient has alerted or attempted to alert the doctor to the problem, in the history taking, in a complaint about unusually severe pain from an experienced mother in labour, in a hunch prior to labour that something is not right with the unborn baby. Alternatively, the clues may arise from other members of the team, the nursing staff, the midwife, or even a relative. Sometimes the patient may not be able to express their concerns or fears, or that they do not understand what is being explained to them. A doctor who listens has greater prospects of detecting and averting problems or misunderstandings and generating patient trust.

Summary of the law and practice relating to consent

+ Valid consent must be obtained before starting treatment or physically examining a patient.
+ Failure to obtain valid consent will expose the doctor to legal liability for negligence and possibly also assault, and to disciplinary action by their professional body.
+ Where a patient suffers harm through a failure to provide sufficient information to allow the patient to give informed consent the doctor may be exposed to a negligence claim for damages.

- For consent to be valid it must be given by a patient with the mental capacity to understand the nature of the proposed treatment and on the basis of sufficient information to make an informed choice.

- The duty to give adequate information is judged in the same way as treatment is judged, i.e. whether the information given complied with the practice of a responsible body of medical opinion.

- Material or significant risks must be disclosed to the patient and balanced with the benefits of the proposed procedure and the risks of not having the proposed treatment.

- All specific questions asked by the patient should be answered truthfully and fully.

- The fact that a patient might be upset by certain information is not a valid excuse for withholding it.

- A choice that is considered unreasonable or irrational by the doctor does not necessarily mean that the patient does not have the appropriate mental capacity. As long as the patient understands the choice they are making they have the right to make that decision.

- If in doubt as to an adult's capacity to understand, then an assessment of that adult's mental capacity should be carried out to determine whether the patient is capable of giving consent.

- For consent to be valid it must be given voluntarily without coercion.

- For most procedures it is not strictly necessary for consent to be given in writing, but it is good practice to have written evidence of the patient's consent.

- Consent remains valid until it is withdrawn by the patient.

- If relevant new information is received by the doctor between the consent being given and the procedure taking place good practice dictates that the patient is informed and their consent confirmed.

- Where an adult is incapable of giving consent the test to be applied is the patient's best interests.

- Nobody can legally give consent for another adult without capacity, although it may be advisable to seek the agreement of other family members to treatment to be carried out in accordance with the patient's best interests.

- Where treatment is carried out under the patient's best interests because they are unable to consent it must be restricted to treatment that is strictly necessary until such time as the patient recovers their capacity. In certain cases the intervention of the court may need to be sought.

- Young people aged 16 or over are entitled to give consent to medical treatment subject to the normal requirements for validity. Refusal to give consent to necessary procedures may be overruled by a parent if the treatment that has been refused is in the child's best interests or welfare.

- Children under the age of 16 may be competent (often referred to as 'Gillick competence') to give or deny consent regardless of their parent's views depending on their maturity and mental capacity. Refusal may be overruled in the case of necessary treatment in the child's best interests as above. In sensitive cases the court's intervention may be needed.

- Where a child does not have capacity to consent that consent can be given by a parent (or someone with parental responsibility) or by the court on the basis of the child's best interests.

- NB in cases of mental disorder different rules apply in accordance with the Mental Health Act 1983.

For a comprehensive guide to the law relating to medical negligence, see *Medical Negligence* (1994) Powers and Harris, Butterworths Law. Department of Health guidance on consent is contained in the DoH publication, *Reference Guide to Consent for Examination or Treatment*.

References

Powers, M.J. & Harris, N.H. (1994). *Medical Negligence*. Oxford: Butterworths.

Reference Guide to Consent for Examination or Treatment. (2001). London: Department of Health.

Taylor, K. (1995). *The Ethics of Caring*. Santa Cruz, CA: Hanford Mead.

Lord Woolf. (1996). *Access to Civil Justice (Final Report)*. Department for Constitutional Affairs.

Chapter 15

Maintaining a balance

Peter Maguire and Carolyn Pitceathly

Summary

Medicine is a worthwhile and personally rewarding profession providing doctors strive to avoid some pitfalls and maintain an appropriate balance between their professional and personal lives. This chapter examines the demands of medical practice, common pitfalls such as unrealistic expectations, needing to appear in control, lack of personal boundaries and poor choice of posts and suggests solutions to enable doctors to cope effectively. Practical tips for junior doctors are found in the appendix to this chapter.

The demands of medicine

Medicine is a very demanding profession, both physically and emotionally. Doctors still work longer hours than other sectors of society. They have to deal with more seriously ill patients because acute beds are in shorter supply and admission thresholds are greater. Patient stays are shorter and it is harder to find adequate time and privacy to talk with them.

While much of doctors' time is spent in providing routine care they are frequently faced with crises and life-threatening emergencies. Dealing with terminally ill patients, relatives of patients who have died suddenly and unexpectedly, and those who are complaining are situations perceived as particularly stressful. Other communication tasks considered difficult include breaking bad news, handling very distressed or angry patients and relatives and patients with difficult personalities.

A key issue is how doctors can cope effectively with those demands and yet maintain a satisfactory balance between medicine and their personal lives. To achieve this goal they must avoid common pitfalls and adopt useful coping strategies.

Common pitfalls and solutions

Unrealistic expectations

The high public expectations that modern medicine is curative can make it hard for doctors to accept a more sobering reality, that many diseases are chronic, degenerative and potentially fatal despite their best efforts. Those doctors who are unrealistic, especially those who are perfectionists in their outlook, will be subject to repeated disappointments, may begin to feel guilty, inadequate and doubt their own worth as clinicians.

Doctors need to take an objective look at what can be realistically achieved, accept this, and be willing to convey this to patients and relatives. For example, in situations where an illness is likely to shorten a patient's life or be chronic and disabling, a doctor's primary aim may change from finding curative treatments to helping patients manage the effects of the illness and achieve optimal quality of life. The doctor who is able to work alongside patients to re-define goals in this way can retain a sense of optimism and satisfaction in the care he offers to patients and their families rather than be dogged by feelings of disappointment and failure.

Doctors may also be intolerant of genuine errors made by themselves or colleagues. They need to realize that mistakes will occur. The key is to learn from them and ensure that they do not happen again.

Internet and other resources mean that patients often research their illnesses and possible treatments intensively. If doctors feel they should 'know everything' an assertive and informed patient may leave them feeling wrong-footed and even intimidated. It is unrealistic for any doctor to be always totally up-to-date and informed. Doctors should have no qualms about expressing interest and taking patients' ideas seriously, if they seem realistic.

The reality may be that other effective treatments are available but cost or individual patients' personal or disease characteristics mean they cannot be offered. Doctors in these situations may feel responsible for failing their patients. The doctor should not take personal responsibility for political or financial factors that are beyond their control. To tell patients honestly why a particular treatment is unavailable or inappropriate shows respect for the patient. The patient with relevant information may be empowered to make a complaint through the appropriate channels or begin to take the reality of their situation on board and accept it.

Needing to appear in control

Refusing to acknowledge strong feelings such as distress, frustration, anger and grief that have been provoked by patients, relatives or colleagues is unhelpful and leads eventually to burnout. Yet many doctors fear that showing and talking about feelings will cause colleagues to label them as 'inadequate' and 'poor copers'.

For the doctors' own psychological health it is key that they acknowledge their feelings and consider what triggered them. They should be willing to talk to like-minded colleagues about it over lunch or in the pub. They will then find such experiences are common and can share ideas on how to manage them.

If they find certain situations, e.g. loss, continue to provoke strong feelings they should consider if these are tapping into losses of their own, in the present or past. If they are they should think about seeing a counsellor.

Sometimes, doctors find themselves expressing feelings in front of patients or relatives, such as crying or being angry because they so empathize with their situation. This is appropriate but it also helps to acknowledge this by saying 'your situation is very distressing. It's got me in tears too'. Patients and relatives will respect this so long as it does not hinder decision making.

Masking emotional distress is unhelpful to doctors' psychological health. It also invites others to have unrealistic expectations of what pressures and workloads doctors can sustain. Only if doctors are willing to share the physical, social, emotional and psychological impacts of their jobs with each other will the culture of 'appearing to cope' change to allow a more open, mutually respectful and supportive culture to develop.

Lack of personal boundaries

Doctors are expected to be able to empathize with patients' predicaments but some get overinvolved. They spend much more time than usual with an individual patient and may even agree to be phoned out of hours. They may also promise outcomes they cannot deliver. This can lead to patients feeling misled, becoming very angry and be a source of much stress. Often patients themselves realize that being too close to their doctor is a disadvantage. For example, one cancer patient who played golf with his doctor, commented that the consultant 'joked' with him about his condition. This effectively prevented him from talking about his worries and concerns because he too felt he must be light-hearted. Similarly, the doctor phoned him with results at home at times when he was unprepared for receiving bad news. To the doctor, holding news until the next clinic, about someone he liked and respected as a friend, felt intolerable. However close the doctor feels to a patient socially or emotionally it is important for both that he maintain professional boundaries or passes the patient on to a colleague.

When boundaries become blurred doctors need to reflect on what their feelings are for the patient. Does the patient remind them of someone important to them in their current or previous life? Are they striving so hard because they loved or love that person? Or are they trying to compensate for negative feelings? Often, such personal reflection is sufficient to encourage doctors to re-establish boundaries. If they cannot, they should seek advice from a colleague or counsellor, especially if overinvolvement comes to represent a pattern of behaviour.

Underinvolvement

Doctors may begin to feel guilty and stressed because they realize they are avoiding patients, for example, those who are dying. Their visits become brief and infrequent. This may be a form of 'self-preservation' because they are feeling overloaded by particularly difficult patients or distressing situations at home or at work. They should acknowledge this, consider what the reasons might be, talk to colleagues or a counsellor. To avoid confronting the problem directly leads to ever increasing guilt and additional stress.

Failure to observe limits

Some doctors wrongly believe that they should be able to deal with all the clinical problems they encounter, even though they have had insufficient experience. This carries the risk of serious mistakes being made and consequent criticism. So, doctors must analyse their clinical strengths and limitations. If in doubt about their ability to deal with a specific situation they should not be afraid to ask for help. Any reasonable senior colleague will be happy to respond. If not asked, they will not be impressed by the young doctors' clinical judgement. Trying to appear more competent and 'pretending' to know leads to mismanagement of patients, complaints from patients and relatives and intolerable levels of anxiety for the doctor.

Similar caveats apply to very distressed, anxious, depressed, psychotic or suicidal patients. Doctors should seek to refer on these patients to a counsellor or psychiatrist or clinical psychologist if and when they feel out of their depth.

Allowing medicine to dominate their lives

It is all too easy for doctors to argue that their prime duty is to their patients rather than themselves and their families. They are then at risk of increasing stress, physical and mental fatigue, burnout and disenfranchisement from their families. To survive, they must strive to find a balance.

Effective strategies including taking regular time out for relaxation and recovery and having other interests that are enjoyable, absorbing and put medicine in perspective. Having friendships with people outside medicine also aids this process. Being able to say no to extra demands is crucial. Instead, every effort should be made to maintain interests in medicine by taking and using study leave to maximal effect. This will also allow any perceived weaknesses to be worked on and should be enjoyable and stimulating.

Poor choice of posts

Some doctors opt for posts they know they are going to find difficult. They are trying to prove to themselves they really can cope with the pressures despite previous adverse experiences. Such counter-phobic behaviour causes immense stress and can lead to depression. Doctors should, therefore, discuss their future job choices with a consultant or tutor who knows them well and be willing to abide by their advice.

Conclusions

Medicine is a worthwhile and personally rewarding profession providing doctors strive to avoid these pitfalls and maintain an appropriate balance between their professional and personal lives.

We have considered what doctors can do to 'maintain a balance' personally. However, doctors cannot do this alone. Part of achieving a balance involves making use of opportunities for training and personal development with peers and colleagues. There must also be an onus on employers and seniors to keep lines of communication open, to be aware of the demands and pressures on doctors and listen both to their difficulties and to their ideas for resolving problems.

Postscript: Practical tips for junior doctors on maintaining a balance

Catherine Hood and Elisabeth Macdonald

Junior medical staff often feel caught in the middle, apparently responsible to everyone: nurses, senior doctors, patients and relatives. If you do not learn how to cope successfully with these demands you can end up disheartened and resentful at a time that should be engrossing and fulfilling. Here are some practical pointers to help keep your head above water.

- Be courteously decisive with patients and colleagues.

- Remember you are an important part of the team.

- There are only two emergency situations requiring immediate response: a cardiac arrest and a distressed relative.

- Assess the importance of what you are being called for. Don't feel embarrassed to say if you have been working non-stop 'I am just going to have my lunch and I will be back in half an hour'. And do come back in half an hour. Other staff will soon learn that you mean what you say.

- There is always time for a quick meal or visit to the loo. You will return refreshed.

- Learn to be good at crisis management.

- Learn to delegate to ward clerks.

- Learn to work well with nursing staff. Learn to be a good team player. Everyone likes to be asked to be involved. Delegate where possible.

- Don't give all the time.

- Learn what help is available. For example, make contact with the palliative care team, the infection control team and the stoma care nurse. Use their advice.

- Emphasize the realistic. Don't offer the unattainable.

- If you 'break down' don't be ashamed. We have all done it. Take a deep breath. Regain your composure and carry on. Your empathy will be respected as long as you then act effectively.

- Remain calm and collected. Do not over-react and do not panic.

- At the end of the day ask yourself: 'Do I really need to do this now, at nine o'clock at night?'

- Go home or go to the pub with a friend. You will be much more efficient at the same task in the morning.

- Keep in touch with non-medical friends.

- Do not allow medicine to come between you and your family.

- Remember, important as you are, you are not indispensable. Take your holiday and your study leave.

- Get on the plane and forget your work for a while. You will be a better doctor for the break.

Chapter 16

Conclusions and future directions

Elisabeth Macdonald

Summary

The doctor–patient relationship is evolving and this chapter looks at the influence of the Internet on this interaction and the different relationship models that may evolve to change fundamentally the types of communication between patient and professional. Useful sources of Internet information are included.

The influence of computer technology on the doctor–patient relationship

Already there is evidence that the doctor–patient relationship is evolving. In whichever way this relationship develops, good communication with the patient will remain pivotal. Already the influence of the Internet can be detected in the medical arena. Although still quite a complex maze of information the internet is already making available knowledge that in the past people have only been able to access through and with the cooperation of the medical profession. This Internet-based knowledge may affect the doctor–patient interaction in a number of ways. Knowledge can help patients prepare for their doctor's visit giving them insight into their clinical situation and facilitating the development of 'activated' patients. Information gained from the Internet may enhance the efficiency of the doctor patient relationship and possibly even save time for the doctor who may no longer have to explain fundamental issues if the patient comes to the visit better prepared. Doctors of course may still suggest where the patient looks for information and in this sense doctors may still 'prescribe' this sphere of patient knowledge.

In the future computer technology may enable doctors and patients to make better diagnoses possibly using specific diagnostic computer programs. This may help to relieve the stress of uncertainty in not knowing what is wrong with the patient. On the other hand, such information may appear simplistic and overoptimistic. It will still fall to the doctor to explain the uncertainties of scientific data in the patient's specific circumstances.

Computer technology could also lead to enhanced co-operation between the doctor and patient. The computer placed in the examination room may give an opportunity for the doctor and patient to collaborate, for example, consulting appropriate websites together. Alternatively, new horizons in telemedicine may facilitate 'virtual outreach' consultations in geographically remote areas with poor access to conventional services.

Currently, doctors act in a sense as a messenger bringing information about the patient's condition to the individual. At the moment doctors are not always receptive to Internet information being brought up during a consultation but there are indications that this state of affairs is changing, at least in the USA. Online health information seekers reported that they discussed the information they found with a doctor or other health-care professional in 37% of cases and of those who talked to an expert 79% said their doctor was interested in the information they found online (Fox and Rainie 2002). Some doctors may feel that this is a challenge to their authority but such a challenge should be viewed as healthy.

Doctors have so far been resistant to communicating with patients via e-mail. Hesitation stems from an anticipation that this will be too time-consuming and threaten confidentiality. However, a carefully prepared set of answers to frequently asked questions, adapted for the individual, could in fact save time during consultations.

Health searchers seem to look for specific answers to targeted questions and appear generally cautious about making decisions based on the information they find without professional corroboration. The ease of using the Internet and the abundance of health information online does not yet seem to be fundamentally changing their approach to health care.

Internet support groups

One new phenomenon, however, has come about enabling those with a specific interest or in this case a specific diagnosis or health problem to create Internet support groups. The revolution in communication and knowledge exchange has facilitated supportive networks or 'virtual communities'. (Powell *et al.* 2003). In the sphere of health problems peer-to-peer support dispenses with traditional barriers and online anonymity can be helpful for those with embarrassing or stigmatizing conditions. Virtual communities supplement the traditional professional relationships and can facilitate the development of well-informed networks with wide perspectives and broad experience of a shared health problem. For example, people suffering from AIDS or HIV infection have created their own support network. These communities can work in tandem with traditional health centres.

In parallel with these virtual communities there has also developed the phenomenon of 'online patient helpers'. For example, a non-smoking Internet expert who developed lung cancer and used her expertise to locate a centre where she could be successfully treated, has set up a website to help those with a similar problem (Ferguson 2000).

Future relationships

Given the new Internet dimension what model may best describe the future relationship between doctor and patient? Wendy Levinson has described three potential models (Levinson 2002).

1. *Citizen model.* This model describes a collaborative partnership with responsibilities incumbent upon both sides. Doctor and patient act as partners in a contract of mutual responsibility. The patient has the right to care at reasonable cost but equally has the responsibility of behaving reasonably in terms of life-style and compliance with an agreed management plan.

2. *Doctor as navigator.* Following the continuing information revolution the role of the doctor may evolve into one more of an Internet navigator guiding the patient in pursuit of appropriate and relevant information concerning his or her condition.

3. *Business model.* This possible development foresees doctors employed by managers to care for customers. This model, which some may argue already reflects some aspects of the employment of the medical profession in the National Health Service, assumes a fundamental change in the professional ethic of the medical professions.

Some clues to the future development of the doctor–patient relationship may be found in what are described as VIP services available in the USA. Under this model the doctor is retained on a 24-hour basis to deliver navigator guidance and health care to an individual employer. This personal service is of course not new to the very wealthy and has been the norm for Royal households over many centuries. It is amusing to reflect that in China during the Ming dynasty, a doctor's pay was stopped when the patient became ill!

Further developments in professional training are foreshadowed elsewhere in the world. 'Skills laboratories', for example, are common in Israel. These provide a teaching and training environment for both the nursing and medical professions together to learn both practical and communication skills in a specific area of medicine. The further development of team-working, and with it a reappraisal of traditional demarcation of training and responsibilities can only improve communication and patient care.

References

Ferguson, T. (2000). On-line patient helpers and physicians working together: a new partnership for high quality health care. *British Medical Journal,* **321**, 1129–32.

Fox, S., Rainie (2002). *Vital Decisions: How Internet users decide what information to trust when they or their loved-ones are sick.* www.pewinternet.org/reports/pdfs/PIP_Health_Report.pdf

Levinson, W. (2002). The future patient and the doctor-patient relationship. *Plenary session: International Conference on Communication in Healthcare,* Warwick 20 September 2002.

Powell, J.A., Darvell, M., Gray, J.A.M. (2003). The doctor, the patient and the world-wide web: how the internet is changing healthcare. *Journal of the Royal Society of Medicine*, **96**, 74–6.

Useful internet addresses

The following list of websites may be useful as a starting point for consumers/patients but also provide doctors with a basic starting point to find specific information sources to recommend in their own specific specialty.

Database of Individual Patient Experience (http://www.dipex.org). A collection, so far limited but expanding, of patients' actual experiences for the benefit of those with similar problems.

MEDLINEPlus (http://www.medlineplus.gov). A general health information finding tool produced by the national library of medicine.

Healthfinder (http://www.healthfinder.gov). From the US Department of Health and Human Services.

The Medical Library Association's 'Top Ten' list (http://www.mlanet.org/resources/medspeak/topten.html). This is a useful device with a highly selective list of quality health information sites trusted by medical librarians.

Web pages for young people to access

http://www.childrenfirst.nhs.uk

http://www.faculty.fairfield.edu/fleitas/contents.html

http://www.teenagehealthfreak.org

http://www.epilepsy.org.uk/kids

Editor's webpage for information and feedback

http://www.dr_elisabeth_macdonald.co.uk

Appendix I

Transcripts of useful illustrative conversations

Catherine Hood and Elisabeth Macdonald

Summary

This appendix contains sample conversations on the following topics: (1) handling an angry patient; (2) breaking the news of recurrence of cancer; (3) discussing cardiopulmonary resuscitation; (4) taking a sexual history; (5) taking a history of abdominal pain (raising relevant sexual issues); (6) breaking the news of an unexpected death; (7) differences of opinion over treatment. This section of the book contains sample conversations between doctors of different clinical backgrounds and their patients. The aim is to give, by example, some ideas for phraseology and approach that may be of practical help. These conversations draw on the experience of senior clinicians who have many years practice of engaging patients in discussion about serious health issues. The conversations chosen represent not only some of the most difficult or distressing topics in medicine but most of them are conversations that may devolve to quite junior doctors in circumstances such as evening or weekend shifts.

These conversations have evolved in two ways. Some clinicians have reproduced a typical conversation, which they have had in the past with many patients presenting a specific clinical problem. In these examples the doctor has imagined a conversation with a typical patient or family member and has reproduced the kind of conversation with which the clinician is very familiar. These are termed 'representative' conversations (conversations 3 and 7).

The second group of conversations result from recordings of senior clinicians discussing a specific problem with an actor or actress impersonating a patient with this clinical problem. These are termed 'enacted' conversations. In preparation for these consultations both the patient and the doctor were provided with a written clinical scenario to provide background to the conversation. The actors participating in these discussions have extensive experience in similar role-play especially helping with communication skills in business and industry. Role-play is seen as an effective way of demonstrating communication skills as well as teaching these skills. The use of specially trained actors to play such roles as customers, staff or interview candidates is now widely used as a powerful methodology to help tackle 'people' issues in the workplace or train managers in media skills.

These conversations were taped on audiocassette (with a backup recorder in case of machine failure). The taped conversations were then transcribed and verified with the participating clinicians. In each case a commentary is added alongside the exchange analysing the techniques and phraseology that had been recorded and the underlying motivation and a short summary follows.

The principal difficulty with this technique is that each conversation probably lasted longer than a truly typical conversation and covered more topics in greater depth than most patients can digest in similar circumstances. As we have observed many important conversations start with the need to impart one major piece of 'bad news' such as a serious diagnosis. This fact will often cause the patient distress and mean that he or she is unable to concentrate on any of the subsequent dialogue. Effective communicators allow for this eventuality by arranging a series of meetings rather than one alone. Often many of the topics discussed would emerge over a series of conversations and often with nursing staff and counsellors as well as medical staff.

The major advantage of this technique was that it made available the considerable experience and skill that each clinician has developed over their career without prejudicing the privacy and trust of actual patients undergoing these very difficult experiences.

Conversation 1: handling the angry patient (enacted)

Background to anger

There are many reasons for patients to react with anger to doctors. Some of these are a normal level of anger, which is understandable when people are under stress and there are delays or mistakes that leave a patient feeling victimized, and without redress.

On the other hand there are some naturally angry people whose normal response to life is anger. If possible this type of angry response needs to be identified by healthcare workers and the problem confronted. It needs to be pointed out that this behaviour is not compatible with care.

However, the anger that we are seeking to demonstrate in this conversation is of a more pathological nature. This anger is usually associated with underlying distress and may have its origin in severe past problems. These may have arisen as a result of family problems and are worst in cases of patients who have previously suffered child abuse. The reaction may date back to early life and resentment of a person in authority. This person who previously caused distress may appear embodied in the authoritarian person of a doctor. Such patients are frightened that a person in authority is doing something to them that is not in the patient's control.

Case history

For the purposes of this conversation the patient we have in mind is a 50-year-old female patient who presented to her GP with what she felt was a lump in the breast. The GP failed to examine her properly and brushed aside her anxiety. She returned on several occasions to see him and finally in frustration he referred her to the local breast clinic. The surgeon in the breast clinic examined her, arranged investigations and these suggested that the lump was benign. The patient returned several times to the clinic asking that the lump be removed because she was not comfortable allowing the lump to remain in the breast. Eventually, the lump was removed and did in fact prove to be a malignant growth. The surgeon was exasperated to have been proved wrong and treated her with discourtesy. Postoperatively she developed a wound infection and she required treatment with antibiotics. The wound healed slowly and she was left with ugly scaring so that the cosmetic result of her surgery is unsatisfactory.

The patient felt that she had been unlucky at every stage and that her future survival was prejudiced by the delay in removing her lump.

In the past she had severe difficulties relating to her family. Her parents were very cool towards her and were unsupportive of her career preferences. She had an older sister who was both better looking and more intelligent and her parents favoured her sister at the expense of the patient. In seeking affection the patient had made a precipitous and unhappy marriage. She is, however, a Roman Catholic and does not feel she should divorce.

Her anger at all this past distress and current fear is manifest in anger at receptionists when there is any delay in her being seen, anger at nurses whom she regards as clumsy and unprofessional and especially anger at doctors who have subjected her to delay, rudeness and unsympathetic handling. Much of her anger is reasonable in the circumstances but because of her difficult personal history the anger becomes disproportionate and prevents her reaching the support she needs.

Transcript of conversation 1

Doctor: Thank you for coming Christine. Your oncologist suggested that we might usefully get together to talk about some of the problems that you have evidently been having in relation to the treatment for your breast problems. Now she has filled me in on some of the background, that is to say that I know you have breast cancer and I know that you had initial surgery for that breast cancer. She has	**Welcomes the patient and sets the scene. States the reason for the consultation but also acknowledges early on the difficulties the patient has had in an understanding and non-judgemental way.**

also told me that you have had quite a rough ride with it. I think it would be useful if you could tell me in your own words what the main problems are at the moment.

Patient: I would have thought you would have known that by now. There has been enough information. The problem now is that I have actually got a terrible terrible scar. I have been left with this intense and ugly scarring after being totally sucked over by the whole system.	Responds with anger.
Doctor: Okay. Tell me a bit about that. How did it come to be that there was a terrible scar?	**The doctor doesn't rise to the patient's anger but remains calm. Listens and tries to clarify points of fact.**
Patient: I don't know. Its not my fault. I am not the medical person. I got an infection. Why did I get an infection? I don't know. Why does that happen? . . .	
(Doctor maintains eye contact but pauses)	
Patient: Well I had surgery and then I got an infection after surgery. The wound did not heal properly and I have been left with very ugly scarring.	
Doctor: And what did the surgeon say about that? Is there any prospect of improving on it for example?	**The doctor encourages and allows the patient to talk. The doctor listens and continues to try and clarify the problems the patient has.**
Patient: Why am I here if you haven't even talked to the surgeon.	
Doctor: Well . . . We're not here to solve the problem of the scarring in itself. What your oncologist . . .	**At all times the doctor is clear about the purpose of the consultation.**
Patient: What are you here for? I mean what are we here for then?	
Doctor: To really look at how these problems are impacting on your life and how you're feeling about it and	
Patient: Well how do you imagine they are impacting on my life?	
Doctor: I can't pretend really to know how that might be for you. That is what I would like to discover from you and to see whether there is any way in which the way	**The doctor shows understanding. Again the doctor encourages the patient to tell her story and listens.**

things are for you and how you feel about them can be made better. Perhaps it would be useful if you could just talk me through the situation as it has arisen. How did you first discover that you had a breast problem?

Patient: I examined my breast. I had been told to do that and I found a lump. I went to my GP, its quite simple and my GP said its nothing to worry about, its your glands. His response was like 'your being a hypochondriac' basically. I went home, I didn't feel comfortable with it and I went back again. He wouldn't examine me properly until I was beating on his door saying look, I really need some help, I know something is wrong.

Doctor: What did you think at the time?

The doctor explores the patient's ideas, concerns and feelings rather than just asking questions of medical fact.

Patient: Well I thought it was cancer. I mean I thought the obvious thing. If you find a lump in your breast, you think you've got cancer.

Doctor: Right!

Patient: I didn't think it was glands. He was a pain in the arse. He was being very difficult this doctor anyway. Finally he referred me and then they told me that they would have a look at it, that there was a lump there and that I should have surgery and have it removed. Then they told me it was benign and then it turned out to be malignant. So I was right all along.

Doctor: How did you feel when you discovered that there had been a mistake?

Patient: Its just very difficult. Why doesn't anybody listen to the patient? I mean the arrogance, the arrogance of the medical profession, the arrogance of doctors, the arrogance of the specialist, they assume that they know everything and they don't.

Anger rises again.

Doctor: So how did it make you feel?

Doctor remains calm and continues to ask about her feelings. They are trying to clarify the underlying issues that are underpinning her anger.

Patient: Can't you see, can't you see how it made me feel? I am furious.

Doctor: Right!

Patient: Its my body and I was dismissed. I was made to feel like nothing. Like I was some stupid housewife who didn't know anything about her own body or had no medical knowledge at all.

The space created by the doctor allows the patient to express her anger and get it off her chest.

Doctor: Clearly you were right. What did the surgeons say to you when the mistake was evident?

The doctor acknowledges her anger and shows empathy. In doing so the patient knows the doctor has listened to her complaint. The doctor remains calm and doesn't rise to her anger.

Patient: Oh. Well actually he was bloody rude! His reaction was unbelievable. It was like he was furious that he had been caught out. Because he said it was benign and it was malignant. He got it wrong.

Doctor: Right!

Patient: He got it wrong and he couldn't handle it. They're so arrogant surgeons, I don't know who they think they are. I mean they wander around in bow ties and grey hair with a load of people around them thinking that they're God and actually they got it wrong and then they can't handle it.

Doctor: Did he explain how the mistake had happened? Did you understand?

The doctor doesn't get drawn into a discussion about blame. A non-judgemental attitude is maintained throughout.

Patient: No, he didn't explain anything to me.

Doctor: Right. So it is something of a mystery to you how this mistake arose?

Summarizes what they have heard and checks it back with the patient.

Patient: Yes and if it hadn't been for me being persistent the cancer could have spread everywhere. As it happens it may still do. Because I had to wait so long to actually get any treatment.

Doctor: How long did you have to wait?

Patient: Oh God, I don't know, about 9 months from start to finish I think.

Doctor: What do you feel about that?	**Continues to explore and so draw out the patients anxieties.**
Patient: I feel insane. Its my life. I mean how do you think I feel?	
Doctor: What is your worry about what happened in those 9 months?	
Patient: Surely you would know the answer to that question. I don't know why you're asking me.	
Doctor: Well for every woman or for every individual it may be different. People have different sets of worries. They have different anxieties. They have different priorities in their life. I am trying not to make any assumptions about what the priorities and issues maybe for you. I mean I am trying to	**Shows understanding and states the reason for asking the questions. Also shows a non-judgemental attitude.**
Patient: I thought life and death was pretty primal wasn't it, I mean they're pretty fundamental. I wouldn't have thought there would be much, you know, variation, shades of grey.	
Doctor: Was the worry for you that the longer you waited the more likely it is that this cancer would be fatal?	**Reflects the possible problem back to the patient.**
Patient: Oh! Well done! Well done!	
Doctor: You clearly are very angry about this.	**Shows empathy.**
Patient: (Angry silence)	
Doctor: Listen. I'm sorry you have had such an awful time. I really do want to help you through this but if I am to find a way to help we really need to put aside the anger you understandably feel and try to deal with some of the other things that are bothering you.	**Demonstrates understanding, acknowledges her concerns as legitimate and apologizes for the situation. Gently explores other possible worries.**
(Silence)	
Doctor: You sound as though you may be very worried about the future. Am I right? Can you bear to tell me a bit more about that?	
(Tears)	
Patient: I don't know who I can talk to; I mean I have been like this all the way along	Through non-judgemental and gentle questioning the patient feels

the line. The main problems have been that I have not been able to get an answer from anyone—Right from the beginning there was no sense that anyone took me seriously. . . . I feel that I don't know where to turn now. I have been left with this terrible scarring; there was an infection after my operation. It has slowly healed but has not healed properly. I don't know why this is and once again nobody can give me an answer. Basically those are the things that are going on with me at the moment.

able to express her frustrations. The dynamic of the consultation has changed as the patient is now more upset and reflective than angry. The doctor has to take more of a lead now.

Doctor: My goodness! Well that is a lot. So not only did you have to deal with knowing you had a cancer, you also had to deal with a sense of, in some way being held accountable or responsible for it. Is that how it felt? That must have been very difficult.

The doctor summarizes the problems and shows empathy and understanding.

Patient: Yes.

Doctor: How do you feel when you look in the mirror?

The doctor explores another potential area of concern.

Patient: I feel disfigured. I don't feel like a woman. I feel ugly and deformed and sad.

Doctor: Tell me who is at home?

Patient: My husband and the kids.

Doctor: How has your husband responded to all this?

Patient: Well in some ways okay. In other ways he doesn't like looking at me. He thinks its revolting.

Doctor: What, the scar? Really?

Patient: He just finds it physically . . . .

Doctor: Is he squeamish? Is one of your worries that he may no longer find you attractive?

Doctor reflects another possible concern with the patient.

Patient: Yes of course. I don't think he does.

Doctor: You mean since the surgery?

Patient: Yes

Doctor: What makes you think that?

Patient: He doesn't come near me. I can just tell.

Doctor: Before this happened did you have an intimate physical relationship with him?

The doctor makes no assumptions about the nature of her relationship with her husband.

Patient: Yes

Doctor: That hasn't resumed since the surgery.

Patient: No.

Doctor: Would you like to have physical intimacy? Do you feel having been through all this turbulent time do you feel that that is something you want?

Explores her desires.

Patient: I want the closeness.

Doctor: Right. Yes. Are you able to talk to your husband about the various fears and issues that you are describing now? Are you able to confide in him?

Suggests a possible course of action.

Patient: Yeah. We talk about it.

Doctor: Is he the person that you normally share your worries and anxieties with?

Patient: Yes.

Doctor: And this has not changed since this cancer. You are still able to do that?

Patient: I know there are certain things he holds back from me because he does not want to upset me.

Doctor: What do you think he is holding back from you?

Patient: That he finds all this hideous. He does not want to feel like that but he sends out a gut reaction of how he does feel.

Doctor: Do you think that, or does he express that? It can be difficult if those things aren't frankly discussed. It may be that, for example, he is just squeamish and also that he is frightened in some way of forcing himself on you at a time when you are vulnerable. There may be a whole raft of reasons why he is not treating you as a robust, physically healthy sexual woman at the moment. It may have very little to do with the fact that he sees you as unattractive but more to do with the fact that he sees

Doctor tries to separate fears from reality. The doctor suggests possible reasons.

you as vulnerable and rather fragile at the moment.

Patient: Will it ever come back?

For the first time the patient asks for advice.

Doctor: Well, what I would say is that usually it does but it requires perhaps some open dialogue between the two of you about what your respective views are of issues and fears and so forth. There is nothing terribly sexy about cancer, or about the fears of life and death, feeling angry and let down and that you can't trust the doctors and nurses on whom your life depends. These are not things that are likely to make either of you feel terribly sexy and so that level of your relationship perhaps needs to be re-found, having been through this terrible ordeal, which clearly you have both been through from what you are saying. I mean maybe you are inadvertently giving off quite negative vibes about him coming close to you physically if you're in pain or uncomfortable.

The doctor suggests a course of action. The doctor shows understanding of the patient's problems and so demonstrates that they have heard the patient's worries.

Patient: Maybe I am.

Doctor: Do you share a bed?

Patient: Yeah. Well he didn't when I got home because I was up in the night.

Doctor: But you're back in the bed together. Does he see the breast on a regular basis or do you tend to hide it.

The doctor explores the problem further picking up on cues that the patient gives about how she feels.

Patient: I hide it.

Doctor: Has he been involved in the care of the wound at all or . . . .

Patient: No I just thought it was just too much.

Doctor: Have the two of you had the opportunity to talk about what having cancer in a broader sense means to either or both of you.

Patient: No I don't think we have really. I think we have avoided talking about it really because there is too much at stake.

The doctor picks up on this cue the patient has given about a major concern.

Doctor: What does it mean to you?

Patient: It means not being there as a mother for my son.	
Doctor: That must be terrifying. Is that something you fear or something that you believe will happen?	**The doctor shows empathy and understanding and tries to clarify whether this is a true belief or just anxiety.**
Patient: I don't know. I think its both.	
Doctor: What have they said to you about the outlook of this cancer? What have the surgeons, what has your oncologist said to you?	
Patient: They said that the percentage of a full recovery is high and that I should hold on to that, because it is a very common operation to remove lumps in the breast.	

Commentary on conversation 1

This is a lengthy consultation with a consultant. The consultation falls into two parts. At first the patient is extremely angry and the doctor is unable initially to 'reach' the patient in a constructive way. However, the doctor picks up on the fact that the patient is frightened for the future. Most people faced with the thought of death lose their anger and this is replaced by sadness and distress. It is in fact easier to reach across to a distressed patient than an angry one and this point in the interview becomes a 'watershed'.

The second part of the interview demonstrates how the patient can be helped to explore the issues causing most distress and also illustrates how some taboo subjects such as sexual intercourse can be approached in a sensitive and unembarrassed manner.

Conversation 2: a conversation concerning the relapse of cancer 5 years after initial treatment (enacted)

Case history

The patient in this case underwent treatment for breast cancer 5 years ago. She has been seen regularly in the clinic and has felt hopeful for all these years that all is well and there was no further need to worry about her breast cancer. However, over the past few months she has developed pain in her back and has reported this to the clinic. A number of investigations have been done that have revealed that cancer has spread not only to her bones but also to her liver and lungs. In some ways the patient will be shocked and distressed by this news and will fear that her life expectancy is very limited. She will be frightened of what treatment this condition may entail especially chemotherapy with sickness and loss of hair.

Part of her reaction, however, will also indicate that this has been news that she has been anticipating since her initial diagnosis and at some level it is not a surprise. She will be very concerned for the welfare of her husband who has Parkinson's disease and who will require her physical help and support in the future. She is eagerly anticipating the arrival of her first grandchild in about 6 months time and will be very anxious to know whether she will be able to survive long enough to see the grandchild and help in caring for it.

Commentary on conversation 2

The doctor tries to combine a fairly realistic account of the situation with an encouraging message that stresses that the patient and health-care team will be working together and that the outlook is not necessarily as bleak as it initially seems.

Knowing that the patient has come for results the doctor does not waste much time in going over side issues but goes almost immediately to the topic, which is likely to be preoccupying her.

Before breaking the bad news the doctor tries to find out what the patient knows about the situation. This gives the doctor a place from which to start the subsequent explanation. Listening to the patient's response will also give a clue as to what she is expecting the test results to be. Her rapid response here would tend to suggest anxiety and an underlying acceptance that bad news might be on the way.

When giving the news, the doctor starts with a short summary of events. Its better to deliver bad news gently as sudden revelations may result in an exaggerated emotional response from the patient due to shock. Getting the pace right is often a concern when delivering bad news. A simple way to get this right is to remain attentive to the impact the information is having on the patient and the cues that they give to continue. These cues can be verbal, such as questions or non-verbal, e.g. the patient maintains eye contact with the doctor. If the doctor is sensitive to these patient cues and speeds up or slows down accordingly, then the pace is controlled by the patient.

Another concern is how much detail to go into. Again this can be gauged by watching for the cues from the patient. If they start to look distracted or take their eye contact away for a sustained time then the patient is signalling that they need some space and time to digest the information so the doctor should pause. When the patient is ready they will ask a question or resume eye contact as is seen in this dialogue.

Once the patient has been given the news its important to allow them space and time to react before going on with the follow-up.

The doctor remains honest throughout about what to expect but the consultation ends with some measured and realistic reassurance.

Conversation 3: cardiopulmonary resuscitation (CPR) (representative conversation)

What follows are several suggested lines of discussion in circumstances where a patient, for example, in the intensive care unit is felt to be seriously ill, likely to develop an acute medical complication that would require CPR. In the view of the medical team the patient is 'competent' to participate in such a discussion and resuscitation (CPR) would have a moderate chance of success, i.e. would not be 'futile' in a clinical sense (see Chapter 6). Many previous discussions have probably taken place at each stage of the patient's illness and this therefore represents a continuation of previous themes.

These are just short snippets of conversation, any conversation in practice would be guided by the response of the patient.

Snippets of conversations about emergency treatment

Good morning Mr Smith. How are you feeling today?

Doctor listens to patient's symptoms with active suggestions to improve patient comfort.

Mr Smith, I would like to bring you up to date on the latest lab results that we've received and then I'd like to discuss with you one important topic about which I'd like your advice.

This forewarns the patient that there is a serious discussion on the horizon.

The doctor has a discussion with the latest practical details of his management then returns to the topic. The doctor may suggest that Mr Smith have a family member present during the discussion.

. . . . so Mr Smith, you can see we seem to be getting your major problems back under control. Things seem to be stable and we hope that with time things will slowly improve. However, its just possible that sudden serious complications could arise and I would like your advice on how *you* would like us to manage these.

The doctor makes it very clear that the patient's opinion is being sought and that the choice is his to make.

I would like your guidance about how 'active' you would want us to be. For example, you've had a very serious infection and had several courses of antibiotics, which gave you quite a few side-effects but have improved your condition. If the infection comes back would you like us to try these again?

The doctor gives an example that the patient can relate to. This will help him make a decision. The doctor highlights the down sides to treatment, e.g. the side-effects as well as the benefits.

. . . . we know that you've had some trouble your kidneys. One way to deal with this if the kidneys get worse is by considering cleaning the blood with kidney dialysis. I'm not suggesting that this is going to happen but it is a possibility and it would be helpful to know whether you have ever thought about this or whether this treatment is something you would wish to try if it has a possibility of helping. Some people at this stage want us to try whatever treatment is appropriate but others prefer to be left alone and continue with measures to relieve symptoms like pain or thirst.

The doctor explores the patient's ideas and seeks his opinion. The doctor makes it clear that not agreeing to dialysis does not mean that his symptoms won't be eased.

Patient nods

. . . . Although you seem well now we know that you have many health problems. Because of these its possible that you might develop sudden heart or lung problems that require urgent treatment. This treatment would probably entail the need to help your breathing and give you heart massage. You would not be aware of this procedure and would not be conscious so I would prefer your guidance as to whether you would like us to undertake this emergency treatment should problems arise.	**The doctor seeks the patient's opinion.**

Pause for patient response

I would have to say that given all the health problems you have I would estimate that this type of urgent treatment would only have a small chance of success with you.	**Is honest about the chances of success.**

Pause for patient response | **Gives the patient time.**

You may want to discuss this with your family or if you don't want to think about it and would prefer for us as your doctors, with advice from your family, to make these decisions for you, you need only say so and we will be happy to do our best for you should the need arise.	

. . . . . . I realize this is a very difficult and painful discussion and not easy for either of us. What I would suggest is that you think about this for a while or have a chat with your family and let me know what you feel. If you would like to talk this through with one of my colleagues or with the nursing staff I would be very happy to arrange this for you. If on the other hand you don't want to contemplate this any further then I quite understand and we promise to do our best for you. I will come back and see you a bit later and you can tell me what you feel'.	**The doctor acknowledges that this is difficult. Gives the patient time to talk to their family and seek further opinions.**

Commentary on conversation 3

For these important discussions patients are encouraged to have the support of a friend or family member if they wish. This discussion was conducted by a senior member of the team who has some knowledge of the patient his/her situation and their family background. Sufficient time is allotted for the patient to be led slowly and gently through this discussion. If possible this discussion should take place on more than one occasion in order to allow the patient to digest the information given and raise any questions that he/she may choose.

Conversation 4: sex and sexuality; taking a history (enacted)

Background history: the GU clinic

This conversation takes place between a doctor in the genitourinary clinic (GU clinic) and Sue Moore, a journalist whose husband is a civil engineer and travels frequently with his work. Recently, Sue noticed a change in her vaginal discharge. It seemed heavier than normal. She thought it might be thrush so bought some Canestan (antifungal cream) from the chemist after which it settled a little.

About 3 weeks ago she developed cystitis (pain passing urine). She went to see her GP who took a sample of urine and gave her 3 days of antibiotics and her symptoms settled. She has been back to see the GP who has told her she did not have a urine infection. She then told him about the discharge and was referred to the GU clinic.

Mrs Moore has regular sex with her husband and uses a coil for contraception. Her periods are regular but have been a little heavier than usual. She has had no abdominal pain or pain having sex. Her last smear was 18 months ago and normal. She has just had two pregnancies.

She has been married to her husband for 10 years. Five years ago she had a casual one night stand with a man at a conference. Her husband does not know about this.

Transcript of conversation 4

Doctor: Hi its nice to meet you. My name is Dr H . . . , I am one of the doctors here. I wonder if you could tell me what has brought you in to see us today.	**The doctor welcomes the patient and asks an open question about why she is here.**
Patient: Well to be honest I am not quite sure why I am here really. A doctor did this urine test on me to test for cystitis and he gave me some antibiotics and it got better, and when I went back to him he said I didn't have a urine infection at all, and he told me I had got to come here and I don't really know why because it is actually better now.	Gives reason for attendance and hints that she expects or hopes nothing is wrong.
Doctor: Okay have there been any other problems at all.	**Doctor explores further and encourages the patient to say more.**
Patient: Well I did have, before that, I had a discharge and I went to the chemist and got some Canestan cream. You know, I thought that that would be the answer and it did get better after that actually so that is not too bad now really.	

Doctor: So that has gone now would you say?	**Doctor checks and clarifies with the patient.**
Patient: Not completely gone but it is much better than it was.	
Doctor: So how long ago was that that you had the discharge?	**Seeks a time frame for the symptoms.**
Patient: Umh, that would probably be a couple of months ago I should think.	
Doctor: And you thought it might be thrush.	**Doctor picks up on an idea the patient mentioned earlier and reflects it back. This shows the doctor is listening.**
Patient: Yeah that's right.	
Doctor: Is that something you have had in the past?	
Patient: I have actually, yeah, and its usually cleared up alright.	
Doctor: Okay. Then you developed the cystitis about a week ago.	**The doctor encourages the patient to continue with her story.**
Patient: About 3 weeks ago.	
Doctor: Did your GP give you anything for that?	
Patient: Yes he gave me some antibiotics and that seemed to do the trick.	
Doctor: Okay. So you're not really quite sure why you have come to see me. Okay, well have you had any other thoughts about what the discharge might be. Any other things crossed your mind?	**The doctor reflects back the patient's stated expectations of the visit then explores the patient's ideas further.**
Patient: I just assumed it was thrush. You know when I was younger I had it a few times I think and I just thought that's what it was.	
Doctor: Well it might well have been thrush but obviously there are some other things that can cause discharge, other infections. So what I would like to do is just ask you a few questions about a bit of background on you to help me to work out whether there is a chance of anything else causing these symptoms.	**The doctor acknowledges the patient's ideas and explains the need for further exploration. The doctor gives a framework for the next part of the consultation so the patient knows she is going to be asked general medical questions.**
Have you got any medical problems at the moment?	

Patient: No.

Doctor: Do you take any medication at all?

Patient: No.

Doctor: Okay. Are you allergic to any medicines?

Patient: No, I don't think so.

Doctor: Okay. When was the first day of your last period?

Patient: I think it was about the middle of July.

Doctor: Are your periods painful at all?

Where appropriate the doctor asks questions that might hint at other causes of her symptoms.

Patient: No.

Doctor: And that hasn't got worse at all?

Patient: No.

Doctor: When was your last cervical smear test?

Patient: I think I had one about 18 months ago and that was fine.

Doctor: Okay. Have you ever had any problems with your smear test before?

Patient: No.

Doctor: Well one of the reasons, I think your GP might have sent you up to us, is for us to see whether there is an infection causing the discharge and the cystitis that you had that hadn't been detected. Sometimes those infections can be sexually transmitted. They may not be but obviously it is one of the things that we need to look into. Because of that I would just like to ask a few questions about your sex life if that is alright with you?

The doctor shares her understanding of why the GP might have suggested this appointment. In doing so she seeks the patient's permission to ask intimate questions and states clearly why she thinks this is necessary.

Patient agrees

When was the last time you had sex?

Patient: Last weekend.

Doctor: Is that a regular partner or casual partner?

The doctor does not assume that the patient is in a stable

relationship. The manner of questioning is non-judgemental.

Patient: Oh I'm married.

Doctor: How long have you been together?

Patient: We have been married about 10 years and we were together a couple years before that.

Doctor: Do you use condoms at all?

Patient: No, I have a coil.

Doctor: When was that fitted?

Patient: Last year.

Doctor: Okay. Any problems with that?

Patient: No.

Doctor: When was the last time you had sex with somebody other than this partner?

Again, the doctor doesn't assume that because the patient is married, she has not had sex with anyone else.

Patient: Well I did once about 5 years ago. I mean my husband doesn't know anything about this. I hope this is in confidence. I did have a one-night stand with somebody.

Doctor: So that was about 5 years ago. Was this just somebody you met or somebody you knew?

The doctor makes it easy for the patient to reveal a casual partner.

Patient: It was just someone I was on a conference with.

Doctor: Okay. Did you use condoms at the time? Can you remember?

Patient: No we didn't.

Doctor: And had you wondered whether that might be the cause of some of the symptoms you have had, or had you made no connection there?

The doctor reflects a possible concern with the patient.

Patient: Well, not 5 years later I wouldn't have thought, no.

The patient reveals that she is not expecting there to be an infection.

Doctor: Alright, well it seems unlikely to be a sexual infection but obviously there is a chance. Often infections can have no symptoms for many months or maybe years, then suddenly cause a problem. What I think would be wise is to

The doctor agrees but explains why an infection cannot be excluded. She suggests the patient has a check-up and seeks the patient's permission.

offer you a full check-up. The examination
is much like having a cervical smear test.
I would insert a speculum into the vagina,
which can feel a little uncomfortable and
then take some swabs using small cotton
buds that you shouldn't feel. I would take
swabs to test for the kind of infections that
might cause your problems, things like
thrush, bacterial vaginosis, which are infections
women just get, but also checking for more
sexually transmitted infections like chlamydia,
gonorrhoea and trichomonas.

Patient: Well I hope it is nothing like that!

Doctor: Does that sound okay?

Patient: Well, we had better do it I suppose.

Doctor: It will certainly give us some more
information to help us sort things out. It will
help us to exclude a lot of things as well.

Commentary on conversation 4

During the conversation the doctor spends a lot of time exploring the patient's ideas
and trying to uncover any anxieties. This information will inform any further discussion should an infection be found.

When taking a sexual history it is important to ask appropriate questions at the right
time. The husband is not mentioned at this stage because the doctor isn't clear what the
diagnosis is. The patient might simply have recurrent *Candida* in which case probing
questions about the husband are inappropriate. Should a diagnosis of a sexually transmitted infection such as gonorrhoea be made then the doctor would explore the patient's
feelings about this. Often patients themselves will bring up the question of where an
infection came from. Its important to be honest about points of fact, e.g. that the infection is sexually transmitted but its not up to the doctor to point the finger of blame.

If the patient suspects that their partner has had another sexual contact the doctor
should deal with the emotional response, provide support and reassure the patient
about the success of treatment.

When taking a sexual history its important to remain non-judgemental and to
make no assumptions about an individual's sex life or sexuality.

Conversation 5: raising issues of sex in hospital; acute abdominal pain (enacted)

Case history

This conversation takes place in the Casualty department between the admitting doctor
and Sally Martin, a housewife and mother who has been sent to hospital because of
pains in her lower abdomen. The pains have been present on and off for a couple of

weeks but now seem to be getting more severe. The pain comes and goes and seems to be focused on the right-hand side. She feels quite sick but has not vomited. Her bowels are normal. Her periods are a little heavy but have been for a while. She has no idea what could be causing this but her GP mentioned that it could be a 'grumbling appendix'.

One of several other possibilities is that she has an ectopic pregnancy.

Transcript of conversation 5

Doctor: Hello I'm one of the doctors looking after you. Can I just ask you a few questions about what has brought you into hospital today?	**Introduction and open question to set the scene.**
Patient: Yes I have got this terrible sort of pain which keeps coming.	Opening statement about symptoms.
Doctor: Can you tell me a bit more about it.	**The doctor asks another open question to encourage the patient to talk.**
Patient: I think it is more kind of on the right side and it is getting worse and it sort of comes and goes all the time and I am really worried about what it is. The doctor thought it might be a grumbling appendix.	The patient talks more about her symptoms and reveals an idea of what it might be.
Doctor: You seem a bit uncertain about that.	**The doctor picks up on her uncertainty about this and reflects it back.**
Patient: Well he wasn't sure. Would that mean I would have to have an operation?	The patient reveals a concern.
Doctor: Well I just want to ask you a few more questions and then we can certainly talk about the options. I mean you said you were quite worried about it. Is there any particular thing you are worried about?	**The doctor acknowledges her concern and explores further.**
Patient: Well you see I have young children. What would happen if I had to go into hospital? Its a bit difficult really.	
Doctor: Have you had any thoughts about what might be causing the pain?	**The doctor asks about the patient's ideas.**
Patient: Well I sort of thought it probably was the appendix. You know I don't really know much about medical things, so I don't really know.	
Doctor: How long have you had the pain for?	**The doctor switches to ask questions about the symptoms.**

Patient: Probably a couple of months now, on and off.

Doctor: Anything bring it on particularly?

Patient: Not that I can think of. No.

Doctor: What do you do when you get the pain?

Patient: Nothing. I mean I've tried indigestion things but it doesn't make any difference so I have to wait for it to go.

Doctor: How long does that take?

Patient: Well it can be a few hours. It is difficult at home with the kids climbing all over me.

Doctor: Can you describe the pain? Is it a sharp pain, a dull pain, a stabbing pain?

Focus

Patient: Well it is sort of sharp but lasts a long time more like an aching pain.

Doctor: So it's achy but gets worse at times. Do you notice any other symptoms with it?

The doctor summarizes what she has heard and checks it with the patient.

Patient: Sometimes I feel a bit sick. I haven't been sick but felt sick.

Doctor: Anything else?

Patient: Not really.

Doctor: Do you think it is generally getting worse?

Patient: Yes definitely getting worse.

Doctor: Okay and that is why your GP sent you here. I just want to ask you a few other questions about you. How have your bowels been? Are they okay?

The doctor lets the patient know that she is going be asked more general questions.

Patient: It's alright. I go to the toilet . . . .

Doctor: So you haven't had any diarrhoea or constipation or . . . .

Patient: No nothing like that.

Doctor: You have never had any problems like this before. Have you ever had any operations before? So you're otherwise quite fit and well.

Patient: Yes I am alright.

Doctor: Are you taking any medication?

Patient: Are you allergic to any medicines?

Doctor: Okay. Well obviously there are a few things this sort of pain could be. It might be the appendix. But there are a few other things we need to exclude. Sometimes you can get pain on the right side and the pain can actually be coming from the ovaries or the uterus as opposed to the bowel, which is where the appendix is. So it could be that there are other things going on. So I would just like to ask a few more questions that might help me to work out where the pain is actually coming from. Obviously one of the things that could cause pain on that right side is an ectopic pregnancy. Is there any chance that you could be pregnant?

The doctor starts to explain the possible diagnoses. The doctor gently raises the possibility of pregnancy.

Patient: Yes I could be.

Doctor: When was your last period?

The doctor explores further.

Patient: I think it was about . . . . . . I am not sure actually, I think I had one in June.

Doctor: And you haven't had one since. Do you think you might have missed a period at all?

Patient: I might have.

Doctor: So there is a possibility. So obviously this is something we ought to bear in mind and we should think of doing a pregnancy test and maybe an ultrasound scan of your tummy.

The doctor suggests action to exclude pregnancy.

Patient: I don't really want another child. I have four already.

The patient gives her thoughts about being pregnant.

Doctor: Well if it is an ectopic pregnancy then it is a pregnancy that is carrying outside the uterus in one of the fallopian tubes, and if that is the case it would involve having an operation to remove the pregnancy. Okay?

The doctor naturally follows on to explain what would be suggested in the event of an ectopic pregnancy. The patient's opinion is sought particularly in the light of her previous concern about an operation.

Patient: Well I know you've got to do whatever needs doing.

Doctor: Well obviously an ectopic is one possibility but sometimes an infection of the fallopian tube can cause pains on the right side as well.	**The doctor follows on to discuss other possible causes of the pain.**
Patient: How would I have got that?	
Doctor: Well sometimes sexually transmitted infections can cause this inflammation of the tubes.	**The doctor is very honest about the types of infections in question.**
Patient: Well I haven't been with anybody else or anything like that.	
Doctor: So you haven't put yourself at any particular risk. But you are sexually active so maybe this is another thing we should check by taking a few swabs. How would you feel about that?	**Having broached the subject the doctor gently explores further and seeks permission to take a few swabs.**

Commentary on conversation 5

In this conversation the doctor gently broaches the possibilities of pregnancy or sexually transmitted infections. Note that the doctor does not take a full sexual history but only asks questions that are relevant to inform the diagnosis. If an infection is discovered then a further, more detailed discussion would have to take place.

Conversation 6: conversation concerning unexpected death (enacted)

Background history

This conversation takes place between a junior doctor attached to the cardiac team and a wife whose husband was brought into the cardiac unit from the golf course where he had been playing golf with his son. She received a phone call from her son the previous afternoon saying that her husband William had felt unwell during the game and thought it was indigestion. He had gone to hospital as a precaution. He had been admitted for a number of tests that had revealed a small heart attack. William had called his wife during the evening from the hospital saying he felt better. He dissuaded her from coming to the hospital immediately saying it was late and there was nowhere for her to stay. During the night his condition deteriorated and the cardiac team had been unable to revive him and he had died. The wife had received a phone call from a nurse saying that his condition was deteriorating and asking her to come to the hospital.

The actress (wife) knows that William has a long history of 'indigestion', a bad cough and was a smoker. He was not a complaining type and was not one to bother his wife or the doctors with his symptoms.

Transcript of conversation 6

Doctor: Hello, are you Mrs Freeman?	**The doctor checks that he is talking to the correct relative and introduces himself and nurse Jones.**
Relative: Oh yes I am, hello. How is he doing? How is he getting on?	
Doctor: I am one of the doctors looking after William and this is staff nurse Jones.	Avoids direct question and keeps in control.
Relative: How's he doing? He wasn't too good when I spoke to him yesterday.	Asks the doctor directly how the patient is.
Doctor: How much do you know about why your husband was admitted?	**The doctor avoids this direct question and keeps control of the consultation. The doctor explores how much the relative knows.**
Relative: Well my son called me to say William wasn't well. They had been playing golf. He was brought into hospital last night in and my son said they were dealing with things and I spoke to my husband and he said that he was okay, not to come over until today really. Then somebody phoned me this morning to say he had taken a turn for the worse so you know, I don't know a lot, I just wondered why they have rushed me in. Did he have a heart attack? I mean I just don't understand. He hasn't had a problem before.	The relative doesn't know many details and is clearly anxious. Her expectation is that he might have had a heart attack. She doesn't reveal any expectation that he might be dead.
Doctor: Your husband came in yesterday and he had problems with what he thought was indigestion.	**The doctor picks up the expectation level of the relative and gently starts to explain events leading up to this encounter.**
Relative: Yes he has always had a lot of that.	
Doctor: Well we did an ECG, a heart test, when he came in which showed that he had what was quite a large heart attack. Now initially everything was fine and we gave him drugs and we sent him up to the ward and he seemed quite comfortable and fine, and obviously that's when you had a chat with him. I popped in to see him during the evening and he was okay. Now unfortunately this morning at around 5 o'clock he did take a turn for the worst.	

Relative: Oh, well can I go and see him?	
Doctor: He started to get some breathlessness and when I went to see him shortly after 5 a.m. his heart attack had become very large and I am afraid to say that the news isn't good. We tried to resuscitate him and make him stable but unfortunately his heart stopped and we couldn't get him back and I'm afraid he died this morning.	**The doctor remains calm and quietly continues.**
Pause	
Relative: He was perfectly alright. I can't believe this. There was nothing wrong with him at all yesterday. I just can't believe it at all. Is my son here?	The relative reacts to the news with disbelief.
Reaction	
Doctor: He is on his way.	
Pause	**The doctor gives the relative time.**
Doctor: I am really sorry. He had such a large heart attack. There was nothing we could do but he wasn't in any pain at the end.	**The doctor empathizes and reassures the relative.**
Relative: I need to go and see my husband.	
Doctor: He is still on the ward and certainly it would be fine for you to go and sit with him if you would like.	
Relative: Yes I want to.	
Doctor: Do you have any questions?	**The doctor invites any questions.**
Relative: No thank you doctor.	
Doctor: Well, I'll leave you with staff nurse Jones who can answer any questions and take you to see William. But if there's anything more you or your son would like to ask me then please ask one of the nurses to give me a call.	

Commentary on conversation 6

This is a common breaking bad news situation. The doctor first checked that he was talking to the correct relative and introduced himself. This is important as mistakes do happen. A nurse has accompanied him, which is important if the doctor is short of time as it allows him to leave the relative with the nurse after the news has been given.

This lady is clearly very anxious and asks the doctor for information. The doctor remains calm and appears to avoid her questions. This might appear bad practice but this lady has expressed no expectation that her husband has died. If the news is given too abruptly the relative is more likely to have an extreme reaction. The doctor doesn't avoid the question, he just opts to break the news more slowly, giving the patient more time to hear what is being said and allowing more time for the doctor to find his words.

Once the news was given the doctor allowed space for the patient to react and then invited questions.

The relative asked to sit with her husband. This is good to offer but it's important to check with the nurses on the ward in advance.

Unfortunately so much sympathy and understanding is conveyed by inflection and the tone of voice that much of the intense and moving emotional message of this interview is lost in transcription.

Conversation 7: handling a difference of opinion over treatment; doctor's unwillingness to treat (representative conversation)

Case history

Senior doctors suggest that one of the most difficult confrontations that can arise occurs when the doctor is reluctant to carry out a procedure for which the patient or family is pressing. One example, in the sphere of renal disease, concerns a patient's demand for his name to be placed on the kidney transplant waiting list when the doctor is clear in his own mind that the patient is a poor candidate for transplantation. The representative conversation that follows exemplifies this problem. In this example a middle aged male patient was grossly overweight, which is a risk factor for the failure of transplantation. National guidelines exist for the addition of patients to a waiting list and the body mass index is known to be closely related to transplant success. The patient was also diabetic with a high risk of occult heart disease and possible cardiac complications postoperatively. The patient therefore needed cardiac assessment as a minimum prerequisite. The specialist felt that the risks of failure were too high and that he would not add the patient to the transplant waiting list for a new kidney unless he both lost weight and the cardiology opinion suggested that the procedure would be cardiologically safe.

Transcript of conversation 7

Patient: Doctor, I absolutely loathe this dialysis business. I'm squeamish and its all so tedious. I know my kidneys are all shot up and my own won't recover. What I need is a new kidney, one that works properly. Can you get me a new one? I've read about transplants. Can't I have one of those?	**Doctor listens to patient's demand.**

Doctor: Unfortunately I don't think that your case is very suitable for a transplant.	**Doctor responds firmly and clearly.**
Patient: Why ever not? I have the same right as anyone else.	
Doctor: Well actually there are good medical reasons not to try it. Firstly, because there is a tremendous shortage of transplant organs, we have a duty only to use these kidneys in circumstances where there is a high likelihood of success. We do know that certain factors make success less likely. For example, we do know that being very overweight, as I'm afraid you are, makes it unlikely that the kidney would last.	**Doctor explains the reasons for his decision and their basis in fairness.**
Secondly, the procedure could be dangerous for you. You have been diabetic for many years and there is a strong chance that there are some underlying heart problems which could make you extremely unwell after the operation and would also lead to failure of the new kidney. I would need to get a cardiologist to see you and give us an opinion about that.	**Doctor explains his concerns for the patient.**
Patient: I don't want to bother with all that. I just know I want a new kidney and I want you to stop messing about and put me on the list.	
Doctor: That's all very well for you. My duty however is to use the small supply of kidneys we have for people who are likely to get most benefit and I can't risk wasting a kidney when someone else is more likely to have a successful and long-lasting benefit. I'm sorry but those are the facts. Perhaps you could lose some weight and we could think again.	**Doctor responds firmly but without anger. He suggests a course of action.**

Commentary on conversation 7

The doctor was clear, firm and fair and having thought the situation through clearly he explained the reasoning in a logical way to the patient but did not give in. It is always difficult not to oversympathize with the patient in front of you to the detriment of other, absent, patients.

References

'Corporate Role-Play', Ashley Callaghan Associates: with especial thanks to Felicity Dean.
Catherine Hood, Ethox, University of Oxford: with especial thanks to Susie Majolier.

Appendix II

A curriculum for communication in medical education

Theo Schofield, on behalf of the steering committee of the RSM Forum on Communication in Healthcare

This document evolved from a Forum on Medical Communication Meeting at the Royal Society of Medicine on 9 November 1999 entitled 'Towards a core curriculum for communication skills learning in medical schools and beyond'. Speakers and contributors to this meeting are listed under acknowledgements.

Background

The ability of doctors to communicate with their patients and with their colleagues is essential for the practice of medicine. There is a growing recognition that some styles of communication are more effective than others, that effective communication can be taught and learnt, and that the ability to communicate should be considered as part of the assessment of clinical competence for medical students and doctors.

The consensus statement issued after the International Conference on Communication in Toronto in 1991 (Simpson *et al.* 1991) summarized the evidence about effective communication, current deficiencies in practice and proven methods of teaching. In 1993 the General Medical Council (GMC 1998) recommended that communication skills should be taught throughout the education of medical students in the UK, and similar statements have been made by the Association of American Medical Colleges (1998) regarding medical education in the USA and Canada.

More recently, the assessment of communication skills has been introduced into the summative assessment of training for general practice and into the examination for Membership of the Royal College of General Practitioners (Tate *et al.* 1999). Other Royal Colleges are also including this assessment as part of their postgraduate examinations.

The General Medical Council's proposals for the revalidation of doctors include communication as a core element to be assessed (GMC 1999). Patients are legitimately expecting more effective communication from their doctors. Greater partnership with patients is one of the aspirations of the NHS plan (DOH 2000). It is likely, therefore, that there will be a demand for continued medical education in this area in the future.

What is less certain, however, is whether there is a consensus about what is to be taught, learnt and assessed under the rubric of 'communication skills'. A published survey in 1998 of communication skills teaching reported considerable progress, but great variability, in UK medical schools (Hargie *et al.* 1998). It could be argued that this leads to healthy diversity between medical schools, but on the other hand a statement of a core curriculum, supported by both evidence and professional consensus has a number of advantages. It could assist those responsible for teaching communication in medical schools to plan their own courses and to make the case for appropriate curriculum time and resources.

A core curriculum can be a guide to individual medical schools and teachers and not be in any way prescriptive. It is 'core' in that it describes the essential elements to be considered, but not necessarily adopted, by all medical schools. It contains statements about:

1. The underlying philosophy of communication in medicine and its learning and teaching.

2. A consideration of the role of medicine in general, and a description of the work of junior hospital doctors for which undergraduate medical education is a preparation.

3. The core competencies required for effective communication in medical practice.

4. Methods of teaching, learning and assessing these competencies.

A core curriculum can also guide the development of assessments for undergraduates and postgraduates, and inform other professional bodies such as the GMC who have responsibilities for medical education. It could be the basis for dialogue with patients, service providers and the government about the importance the profession places on effective communication.

Methods

With these potential advantages in mind the Forum on Communication in Healthcare of the Royal Society of Medicine embarked on the process of defining a core curriculum for communication in medical education. A first step was to learn from the experience of Teachers in Medical Ethics who had undertaken a similar exercise and reported very favourably on the impact they felt such a document could make

(Consensus Group of Teachers of Medical Ethics and Law in UK Medical Schools 1998).

The Forum held three meetings attended by teachers and practitioners in medicine and other health disciplines. At these meetings the concept of a core curriculum was considered and widely supported, and the content discussed. Teachers in medical schools were asked to provide copies of their current programme of communication skills teaching, and 10 curricula were reviewed. A discussion paper was produced and circulated to members of the forum, teachers and Deans in Medical Schools, and other interested parties. Forty-two responses were received. All supported the development of a curriculum as guidance to medical schools, and a number also highlighted its relevance to postgraduate education as well. This document reflects the consensus achieved and the many detailed comments that were made.

Underlying philosophy

The principles that informed the content of the curriculum are that it should:

Reflect the ethical principles of health-care practice

These have been described in a number of ways, for example Beauchamp and Childress (1979) stated four prime facie moral principles: respect for autonomy (the patients rights, particularly to make informed decisions about their health care free of pressure); beneficence (acting in the patient's best interests); non-maleficence (avoiding harm); and justice (or fairness).

The GMC's statement of the Duties of a Doctor (GMC 1995) include:

1. Make the care of your patient your first concern.
2. Treat every patient politely and considerately.
3. Respect patients' dignity and privacy.
4. Listen to patients and respect their views.
5. Give patients information in ways they can understand.
6. Respect the rights of patients to be fully involved in decisions about their care.

These ethical principles should be reflected in the teaching and practice of communication.

Reflect the empirical evidence of the effects of styles of communication on patient outcomes

There is a growing body of evidence that relates certain aspects of communication, for example, understanding the patient and their concerns, sharing information with patients, and involving patients in decisions and in their continued care, with outcomes such as reduction of concerns, symptom relief and health status (Stewart 1995). This evidence demonstrates the links between effective communication and clinical practice and should guide what is to be taught and learnt.

Enable learners to respond to the needs of individual patients

Communication teaching is not about promoting a single style of communication. It should enable the learners to respond appropriately to their individual patients, including those of a different age, gender and culture.

Promote personal and professional development

The ability to communicate effectively depends on the confidence, values and self-awareness of the person. Teaching, and teaching methods, should be selected to be appropriate for the students' stage of development, and designed to promote personal growth and awareness.

Promote reflective practice

Teaching should be the start of life-long learning, and should be designed to develop a willingness to be reflective and to give and receive constructive feedback.

The role of a junior hospital doctor

All teaching is more effective if it is seen as relevant by the learner, and medical students are inevitably focused on their current work with patients and on their assessments. As they progress through medical school they become increasingly aware of the need to prepare for their work as a junior hospital doctor. A curriculum must reflect the needs of doctors and their patients and take account of the role of a junior hospital doctor.

Building relationships with patients

The junior doctor is often the first doctor the patient sees on admission, and has the most frequent contacts with them. They need to be able to establish effective relationships with their patients and their families so that patients feel cared for, listened to, and confident in the treatment and information that they receive.

Information gathering

The ability to 'take a history' is fundamental and is usually understood to mean the gathering of clinical information and its presentation in a structured format. The evidence about patient-centred consulting indicates that this process involves actively listening to the patient's story, and the 'history' needs expanding to include not only understanding the patient's problem, but also their perspective, their ideas, concerns, and their wishes and expectations about their care.

Sharing information

The junior doctor is often the main source of information about diagnosis and management, and this needs to be conveyed in ways that the patient understands and can inform their decisions. Frequently the information is 'bad', in other words it can adversely affect the patient's view of the future, and the ability to do this sensitively is crucial for the patient.

Involving patients in decisions and their care

Recent guidance on Informed Consent (DOH 2001) suggests that for major procedures this should be discussed with more senior doctors who will be, or are trained to, carry out these procedures. However, junior doctors are still involved in discussions about investigations, treatments and care after discharge. Patients expect to be at the least informed about these, and given the opportunity to share or make these decisions themselves.

Communicating with people of diverse backgrounds

Patients have a wide variety of backgrounds and cultures, and are often of a different gender and a very different age from the doctor. Junior doctors need to understand these differences and their implications for communication. Special skills are also required to communicate with children, older people and those with sensory difficulties.

Team care

Junior doctors work as part of teams. They are part of a hierarchy within medicine, and work as colleagues with other health professionals. Understanding, positive attitudes and team-working skills are essential, including respect and willingness to learn from others, and appropriate assertiveness. Doctors also take part in small group discussions and meetings as part of their work, which also require particular skills.

Other methods of communication

Communication via the telephone, the use of medical records and computers, and by Email are all growing in importance. Doctors also need to present their work on ward rounds, at meetings and in writing, and all these skills are part of effective communication.

Self-awareness and survival

Junior doctors work under multiple pressures. Time and workload is reportedly the greatest, but other pressures include the distressing nature of illness, responding to the concerns, fears, and sometimes complaints of patients and their relatives, and working in an environment where resources for patient care and staff support are limited. It is easy to develop maladaptive and uncaring defence mechanisms.

Junior doctors need time management skills, the willingness and ability to give and to receive support, and an awareness of the limitations and boundaries of their role. They also need to be able to acknowledge their own limitations and respond appropriately when things go wrong.

Core competences

In the light of the underlying philosophy and an analysis of the role of the junior doctor the core competences to be learnt and assessed were defined.

Attitudes and values

The learner should be able to demonstrate that they possess appropriate attitudes and values including:

1. Making the care of their patients their first concern.
2. Respect for their patient, their dignity and privacy.
3. Respect for their patient's views and cultural diversity.
4. Respect for the patient's autonomy and right to be involved in decisions about their care.
5. Awareness of their own feelings and limitations.
6. Respect for the professionalism of other team members.
7. Willingness to seek, and to give, appropriate support and feedback.
8. Honesty and openness in their dealings with patients and colleagues.
9. Willingness to acknowledge their limitations and mistakes.
10. Willingness to maintain and improve the quality of their care throughout their professional lifetime.

Patient-centred consulting

The learner should be able to conduct a patient-centred consultation in which they:

1. Define the nature and history of the patient's problem, its aetiology and its effects.
2. Explore the patient's perspective, their personal and social circumstances, and their ideas concerns and expectations.
3. Explain the problem, its prognosis and the options for management in ways that the patient understands.
4. Enable patient's to make choices about their management.
5. Involve patients appropriately in the management of their problem.
6. Use time and resources appropriately.
7. Establish an appropriate relationship with the patient in which the other tasks can be achieved.

Core skills

To achieve patient-centred consultations the learner should be able to demonstrate the ability to:

1. Open a consultation and establish a rapport with the patient.
2. Actively listen to the patient, and recognize and respond to cues.
3. Use open, closed and focused questions appropriately.
4. Retain and interpret information, and generate and test appropriate hypotheses.
5. Clarify and summarize information given by the patient.

6. Give explanations that respond to patient's ideas, are clear, and use appropriate language.

7. Consider options with the patient and enable shared decision making.

8. Involve patients in their management and enhance concordance.

9. Observe and interpret non-verbal communication in the consultation.

10. Respond appropriately to the patient's concern or distress.

11. Demonstrate empathy for the patient.

12. Structure and guide a consultation so that time is used appropriately.

Communication in specific circumstances

The learner should be able to demonstrate the ability to communicate with patients effectively in the specific circumstances that they may encounter, including:

1. Communication with relatives and family groups.

2. Communication with older patients.

3. Communication with children and their parents.

4. Sharing difficult news.

5. Talking to the bereaved.

6. Discussing 'do not resuscitate orders'.

7. Giving advice about life-style and behaviour change.

8. Exploring sex and sexuality.

9. Communicating with patients with sensory impairment or communication difficulties.

10. Communicating with patients with learning difficulties.

11. Communicating with patients with mental health problems.

12. Dealing with complaints, and when things go wrong.

13. Responding to anger and aggression.

14. Recognizing and responding to patients with medically unexplained symptoms.

15. Working with interpreters.

Other aspects of communication

Beyond doctor–patient communication the learner should be able to demonstrate skills in:

1. Teamwork and communication with other team members.

2. Communication in small groups and meetings.

3. Assertiveness.

4. Communication on the telephone.

5. Written communication and recording.

6. Presentation skills.

Knowledge

The learner should demonstrate a knowledge and understanding of:

1. The psychology of interpersonal communication in relation to the doctor–patient relationship.
2. The ethics and legal aspects of the doctor–patient relationship.
3. The social and cultural context of the doctor–patient relationship.
4. The empirical evidence about effective doctor–patient communication.
5. The range of patients' experience and responses to illness.

Approaches to learning

This body of knowledge, skills and attitudes will be taught and learnt in different ways in different medical schools and by different individuals. There is, however, a consensus about some aspects of learning and teaching that is shared, and is based on a substantial body of empirical evidence (DOH 2001).

Communication is a thread that should run through medical education and should be re-visited at each stage of the learner's development

The teaching should be appropriate to that stage and relevant to their other activities and work at the time. How this is planned will vary but it is easy to see how a medical school might choose to include the background knowledge as a preclinical topic, the core skills early in clinical teaching, the special situations during appropriate clinical modules, and other aspects of communication in the period of preparation for PRHO jobs. Some issues such as breaking bad news and somatization may be re-visited again during postgraduate education.

Effective communication should be regarded as a core clinical skill and integrated with clinical teaching

The core skills for conducting a patient-centred consultation, particularly listening, questioning and hypothesis testing, are the skills required to be an effective diagnostician. Students will learn both skills and attitudes from the modelling and reinforcement provided by their clinical teachers. For example, the process of 'clerking patients' and then presenting their histories could promote patient-centred consulting if the learner was always expected to be able to say what the patient understood, what their concerns were, and what their preferences were for treatment. This has implications for teacher development.

Patient centred-consulting is best learnt by learner-centred teaching, and from a variety of teaching methods

These include small group teaching, and opportunities to practise with either real or simulated patients, and to receive feedback from their teachers, their peers and their patients.

Students should be encouraged to learn from their patients and from their colleagues in other disciplines

This can be done informally by being open to feedback, and in more structured sessions that involve patients and members of other disciplines. Team-working skills should be both modelled and taught.

Teaching about communication and the doctor–patient relationship will be enhanced if it involves other disciplines, including ethics, law and the medical humanities

This broad-based approach may help to avoid teaching in communication skills being regarded as learning a set of techniques, but rather seen as an integral part of personal and professional development.

Teaching should be adequately resourced

An effective teaching programme in communication requires trained teachers with the time to teach and to co-ordinate the programme, the involvement and support of clinicians and members of other disciplines, sufficient suitable space for small group teaching, and the money to pay simulated patients for teaching and assessments. There is a growing consensus among teachers of communication about the requirements for the development and implementation of communication skills teaching, and a statement of these was published in 1999 (Makoul and Schofield 1999).

Approaches to assessment

Assessment of effective communication is being developed in medical schools and postgraduate medical education and a variety of methods are being used. There is a consensus about some of the principles that should guide these developments.

1. *Assessment of the ability to communicate effectively is essential at all stages of medicine.* This is to protect patients because it is an essential ingredient of clinical competence, to help students by identifying their learning needs, and to assist teachers, because their teaching will be valued less if it is not assessed.

2. *Assessment should include observation of communication, either with real, or with simulated or standardized patients.* This is labour intensive, even if, as in some places, the patients also act as the assessors. Second-hand assessments of an interview, based on the ability to present an accurate history, do not capture many of the learning objectives that have been described. The clinical content of an interview is distinct from the communication, even if served by it, and each should be assessed specifically.

3. *Assessments should be based on the ability to communicate effectively as well as the performance of particular skills.* This enables students and doctors to develop their own styles and to be judged on their effectiveness, rather than on their conformity to a particular approach, and becomes more important as their experience develops. Effectiveness in a doctor–patient interview can be defined as the achievement

of patient-centred tasks. The assessment of attitudes and communication in other settings, for example with colleagues, may not form part of a summative assessment; however, they can be included in other assessments, for example, end of firm reports.

4. *Assessment should be formative as well as summative, and opportunities for remedial teaching should be available for those who are found to require it.* This reflects the importance of communication, and also the need to protect the needs of both learners and patients.

Conclusions

This appendix is a set of recommendations that are primarily intended to be of value to those responsible for teaching communication in medical schools in the UK. They may also be of interest to other bodies involved in the development of medical education, including the General Medical Council and the Royal Colleges. The core competencies are relevant to medical practice, and may also be included in postgraduate medical education and assessment.

Acknowledgements

This paper is based on the contributions of all those members of the RSM Forum on Communication in Healthcare and teachers in medical schools who attended the workshops and commented on earlier drafts. Jane Kidd, Lorraine Noble, and Debra Nestel commented on all the drafts of the document and contributed many of the references.

Participants' list

Towards a core curriculum
9 November 1999
Communication Healthcare Forum

Dr John Benson
Director of Education
GP Unit, University of Cambridge

Mr Patrick Benson
Shirehall Communications

Dr Julian Bird
Consultant Psyhchiatrist
GKT

Mrs Jan Cambridge
Project Officer
University of Liverpool

Dr Simon Cocksedge
Lecturer in General Practice
University of Manchester

Mrs Penelope Conway
Ethics Co-ordinator
British School of Osteopathy

Dr Jan Van Dalen
University of Maastricht

Mr Gerard Darby
Freelance

Dr Tim Dorhan
Consultant Physician
Salford Royal Hospitals

Mr Phillip Doulton
Director of Com Company
GKT

Dr Al Dowie
Dundee

Dr Iain Duthie
Communication Skills Organiser
Aberdeen University Medical School

Dr Sarah Ford
Research Fellow
Oxford University, Ethox

Dr Elaine Gill
Communication Skills Unit
Guy's King's & St Thomas' Hospital

Dr Peter Haughton
Adviser in Medical Ethics and Law
Guy's Kings & St Thomas' Hospitals

Mr Miriam Hawkins
Project Leader
West Yorkshire Simulated Patients

Dr Catherine Hood
Research Fellow
Ethox, Oxford

Dr Gerry Humphris
Professor In Health Psychology
University of St. Andrews

Pam Iannotti
Undergraduate Co-ordinator
Royal South Hants Hospital

Mrs Rosie Illingworth
Communication Skills Facilitator
University Of Manchester

Dr Sue Kaney
Phase 1 Director Communication Skills
University of Liverpool

Miss Catherine Kennelly
Researcher
College of Health

Claire Kenwood
Consultant Psychiatrist
Royal South Hants Hospital

Dr Jane Kidd
imperial College School of Medicine

Ms Penny Lazarus
Student
Med Human Relations

Dr Paul Lazurus
Lecturer in General Practice
University of Leicester

Dr Margaret Lloyd
Reader in General Practice
Royal Free & University College
 Medical School

Dr Christopher Mallinson

Dr John McMullan

Ms Penny Morris
Assosciate Adviser in CPD
Addenbrookes Hospital

Dr Debra Nestel
Lecturer in Communication Skills
Imperial College

Dr Lorraine Noble
Lecturer in Communication Skills
UCL

Dr Karen Nudgent
Lecturer in Surgery
University of Southampton

Mrs Isobel Nunneley

Ms Bernadette O'Neill
Communication Skills Lecturer
University Hospital Lewisham

Dr Fawzia Rahman
Consultant Paediatrician

Dr Charlotte Rees
Lecturer in Behavioural Sciences
QMC/University of Nottingham

Dr John Rees
Assistant Clinical Dean
Guy's King's & St Thomas' Hospitals

Dr Robbie Robertson
Senior Clinical Tutor
Glasow University

Dr Theo Schofield

Gillian Tierney
Producer
BBC Science

Dr Jonathan Silverman
Director of Communication Studies
Clinical School, Cambridge

Dr Alison Sinclair
Clinical Lecturer
University of Edinburgh

Dr John Skelton
University of Birmingham

Mrs Ann Smith

Dr Naresh Sood
Course Oraniser - VTS Clinical Tutor CME
Nottingham University

Dr John Spencer
Professor of Medical Education in
Primary Health Care
University of Newcastle

Dr Chris Stephens
Southampton General Hospital

Dr Anita Thomas
Dir Med Education
Plymouth

Dr Derek Timmins
Consultant Physician
Royol Liverpool Hospital

Ms Connie Wiskin
University of Birmingham

....

Speakers and chair persons are written in italics.

References

Association of American Medical Colleges. (1998). Learning Objectives for Medical Student Education. Guidelines for Medical Schools. Washington DC: Association of American Medical Colleges.

Beauchamp, T.L., Childress, J.F. (1979). *Principles of Biomedical Ethics.* New York: Oxford University Press.

Consensus Group of Teachers of Medical Ethics and Law in UK Medical Schools. (1998). Teaching medical ethics and law within medical education; a model for the UK core curriculum. *Journal of Medical Ethics,* 24, 188–92.

Department of Health. (2001). *Reference Guide to Consent for Examination or Treatment.* London: DOH.

Department of Health. (2000). *The NHS Plan.* London: DOH.

General Medical Council. (1995). *Good Medical Practice.* London: GMC.

General Medical Council. (1998). *Tomorrow's Doctors.* Recommendations on undergraduate medical education issued by the Education Committee of the General Medical Council in pursuance of Section 5 of the Medical Act 1983. London: GMC.

General Medical Council. (1999). *Performance Procedures a Guide to the Arrangements.* London: GMC.

Hargie, O., Dickson, D., Boohan, M., Hughes, K. (1998). A survey of communication skills training in UK Schools of Medicine: Present practices and prospective proposals. *Medical Education,* 32, 25–34.

Makoul, G., Schofield, T. (1999). Communication teaching and assessment in medical education: an international consensus statement. *Patient Education and Counseling,* 137, 191–5.

Simpson, M., Buckman, R., Stewart, M., Maguire, P., Lipkin, M., Novack, D., Till, J. (1991). Doctor–patient communication: the Toronto consensus statement. *British Medical Journal*, 303, 1385–7.

Stewart, M.A. (1995). Effective physician-patient communication and health outcomes: a review. *Canadian Medical Association Journal*, 152(9), 1423–33.

Tate, P., Foulkes, J., Neighbour, R., Campion, P., Field, S. (1999). Assessing physicians' interpersonal skills via videotaped encounters: a new approach for the Royal College of General Practitioners Membership examination. *Journal of Health Communication*, 4(2), 143–52.

Index

Royal College of General Practitioners
xvi–xvi, 209
Royal Society of Medicine xv, 210

satisfaction, patient
closing phase of consultation 16
first phase of consultation 11, 13
importance of good communication 2, 3
second phase of consultation 14
second opinions 91
security measures 81
senile illnesses 38–9, 105
sensory impairments
children 95
elderly people 103–5
sexuality issues
Afro-Caribbean community 146
Jewish people 143
representative conversation 196–204
see also reproduction and fertility issues
sickle cell anaemia 146
sight problems, elderly patients 105
silence, doctor's use of 8
skills laboratories 180
socio-economic issues 38, 42, 44
multicultural society 132
speech and language therapists 95
spouse see family and friends
stigma of disease 38
cultural issues 133, 139, 146–7
stroke
ethnic minority groups 132
non-compliant adults 102
strong emotions 77–8, 85
anger 80–1
distancing from 78–9
distress 79–80
life support, withdrawal of 55–6
withdrawn patients 81–2
support for colleagues 126–7
support groups for patients 179–80
surgery, patient's perspective 38
syphilis 145

tape recorded consultations 9, 112–13
advantages 113–14
disadvantages 114
teamwork see multiprofessional
communication
teenagers 96, 99–102
telemedicine 179
telephone consultations 109–10
terminology
adolescents 100

cultural issues 131
paediatric medicine 92, 94
tape recorded consultations 114
time management 16–17
garrulous patients 18
reticent patients 18–19
second phase of consultation 14–15
Toronto consensus statement xviii, 209
training, professional 180
transference issues 40
translators, consultations through 110–12
transplant co-ordinators 59, 60, 61
transplants 58–61
Afro-Caribbean community 147
treatment issues, patient's perspective 37–8
trust
in doctor–family relationship 55
in doctor–patient relationship xix–xx
adolescents 100
apologies and errors 152
doctor's perspective 47
eye contact 9
first phase of consultation 12
importance of good communication 2
paediatric medicine 89
reticent patients 18, 19
truth see honesty
tuberculosis 38, 133
Tuskegee Syphilis Experiment 145

uncertainty 47
breaking bad news 71–2
obsessional compulsive patients 84
underinvolved doctors 175
undesirable behaviour, talking about a
colleague's 122–3, 125
confronting the situation 124
preparation 123
resolution 124–5
time and place 123
unexpected death
bereaved people 107
breaking news of 69–71
representative conversation 204–12
Urdu 137
utilitarianism 22

value judgements 21
values, doctors' 213–14
venereal disease 38
VIP services 180
virtual communities 179–80
visual impairment, elderly patients 105
vote for life campaign 59

Printed in the United Kingdom
by Lightning Source UK Ltd.
131455UK00001B/18/P